A Well Made Man

Nuri Muhammad

Printed in the United States of America.
Published by Bashirah House Publishing - First Edition, 2022
Editing: Traci C. Muhammad (Phoenix, AZ)
Transcription: Shareefah Muhammad (Houston, TX)
Cover/Interior/Editing: Rodney 'Asaad' Muhammad (Phoenix, AZ)

Table of Contents

Introduction

To love God is to love your brother: Our duty to one another

Brothers: If God created you "from Himself," that means every one of you is a God, and has God's Divine Nature in you! As David The Psalmist says, "Ye are all gods, children of The Most High God." Now let's get the Bible and Qur'an to back this up!

In the Bible, 1 John, Chapter 4, verses 20-21, it reads: "If a man say, 'I love God,' and hateth his brother, he is a liar: for he that loveth not his brother whom he hath seen, how can he love God whom he hath not seen? And this commandment have we from him, That he who loveth God love his brother also." Let's stop a minute, and look deeper into what John The Apostle is saying. What do you mean "How can you love God Whom you've never seen, and then hate your brother?" Then there is something in your brother that is of God!

So when you hurt your brother, you're hurting your Father! I'm a father, brothers; I've got 9 children, 23 grandchildren, one great-grandchild! And if I ever see my children fighting, it gives me such pain! If you are "God"—not "big God," but a little "God," made as the Bible teaches "in the image and the likeness of God," then Elijah Muhammad said, "Every time I see a Black man, *I'm looking at God." So when I look at you: I don't have to "wait" to see The Father, for I see The Father in you! And when we refer back to what Surah 4, verse 1 says, "O people, keep your duty to your Lord"—so when I see you, I have a duty by you, brother!*

—Honorable Minister Louis Farrakhan

The Return of The Original Man = A Well Made Man

When we are dealing with 'The Return of the Original Man, 'we are not talking about the first man, from trillions of years ago, coming back today himself *physically*. We are not talking about His return as a character, but the return of His character in us! We are dealing with what really makes a man who and what he is—his ***quintessence***, his core, the inner spiritual self. We are not a body with a mind in it. We are a mind with a body wrapped around it. When the wise inquired of Solomon, 'How would you define man? 'He said, "As a man thinketh in his heart, so is he." Solomon did not say, 'As a man weareth, 'or 'As a man driveth, 'or 'As a man liveth in 'The house, the car or the clothes we wear do not define us as men. *A Well Made Man* starts with a Well Made Mind. The Return of the Original Man takes place with the return of the original mind. The original mind is the mind of God. This is why Philippines 2:5 says. 'Let this mind be in you the same mind that was in Christ Jesus. Christ had the mind of God, so he could say when you see me, you see the father. For I am in the father and the father is in me. Why? Jesus underwent a mind transplant! Let this mind be in you…? This means we've been invited to receive the same mind transplant Christ received, making us what is written in Romans 8:17, Joint Heirs with Christ. An Heir is the recipient of an inheritance. Our inheritance is God's Mind. When the process of not being conformed to the ways of this world but being transformed by the renewing of our mid is complete, we become the

God we believe in! ' Our minds have been murdered but our bodies are still in motion. This state makes the Black man, the real walking dead! This is what the "resurrection" of scripture is all about.

Resurrection has been styled as rising from the grave. However, resurrection is not a singular event that takes place when a physical body rises from its burial place in a cemetery. In the book of Job in chapter 7 we find Job being questioned about life after death, Job responds by saying, *"My life is wind and once I go down into the ground I shall come up no more. The eyes that have seen me shall see me no more. The ears that have heard me shall not hear me no more."* Job is clearly saying that when he is gone, he is gone; therefore, The Return of the Original Man is not the return of his body, it is a return of the state of mind that he had prior to his fall.

When we look at the phrase, '*resurrection from the grave*,' we find that within the word '*gravity* 'is the word *grave*. The base word of gravity is grave. What then is gravity? Gravity is the unseen force that exists 6 miles above the planet. It is an invisible force that holds objects down on the surface of the planet. When we think or speak about the resurrection from the grave, we are not thinking or speaking about momma, uncle, auntie or grandma coming up out of a cemetery? No! We are talking about the original people being raised from whatever forces in this world that are holding us down! In the grave could be drugs, alcohol, sex, greed, lust, lies, miseducation, or negative self-defeating commands that have been installed in our thinking from spirit killers, dream snatchers, and the aspiration assassins we've met in our sojourn. Whatever is holding us down, once we successfully overcome it, that is the true resurrection from the grave. Resurrect to Re-Erect. *Erect* means to stand back up. *Re-* means again. To be resurrected is to be stood up again. Again. Again. This means we have to study what we were when we were up, then engage in the process of restoration, that we may be the men we were, before we were hit in the head and left for dead.

Restoration

We learn in the study of restoration, the process of objects returning to their former state or glory, that there are three primary principles, which guide the practice. When an antique dealer wants to bring back a high value object to its original form, no matter if it is a classic car, a painting by one of the great artists of a particular time or a house, these three things are always required. To return or restore something back to original, you need:

A ***Prototype***, A ***Process*** and A ***Proof.***

For example, if I had a two door Cutlass SS and I wanted to restore it to its original state then I would need a prototype that clearly and accurately showed how it looked and functioned in its original form. Once we have a *prototype*, then we can calculate, consider, and compare our version to the original version and go to work with a *process* to turn that which is, back into an accurate mirror *(proof)* of that which was when it was in first made. A house the same way. An Antique, the same way. We are not dealing with returning a car, a house, or an antique back to its original state. We are dealing with The Return of The Original Man; therefore, the question that we must ask is, 'What did the original man look like? 'What is the *prototype*? What is the *process* by which we get to the goal, and who is the *proof* that the process does in fact work? Let's unpack it.

A prototype, the word 'proto 'means "first, foremost or the earliest form of." When Master Fard Muhammad asked the Honorable Elijah Muhammad ten questions and received ten answers, the first one He asked actually gives us the absolute prototype. Master Fard Muhammad asked: ***"Who is the Original Man?"*** If Master Fard Muhammad is asking who is the Original Man, and His Messiah, the Honorable Elijah Muhammad is answering, then this answer gives us a description of what the prototype is made of. The Honorable Elijah Muhammad answered, ***"The Original Man is the Asiatic*** Black man**."** He's the what? And the what? He's ***"the Cream of the Planet Earth***" and he's the what? ***"God of the Universe."*** This then is the prototype and definition of what the Original man *looks* like, *acts* like and *functions* like.

Brothers, in truth, there isn't a woman who upon hearing that definition doesn't say to themselves, 'I need me a man like that, I need me a man that knows how to make something. Knows how to own something! I need a God of the Universe!' The Black woman wants and deserves a man like this; however, there is a process involved. Before a Blackman can be the *God of the Universe*, he must be the God of a planet. Before he can be the God of a planet, he has to be the God of a continent. Before he can be the God of a continent, he must be the God of a country. Before he can be the God of a country, he must be the God of a state, the God of a city, the God of a hood, the God of a house, and the God of self. When a man learns how to establish and maintain freedom, justice, equality, harmony, and balance within *himself*, then it is only a matter of time before we as men begin to say, "Be and it is!" All Praises are due to Allah (God).

The Honorable Elijah Muhammad described us as the Asiatic Black man. In this world when we think of Asiatic, we think of Korean, Chinese, and Japanese. This is not the Asiatic that the Honorable Elijah Muhammad is drawing our attention to, because at one point the entire Earth was called Asia. If you are diligent students, you can find maps that have survived to this day, where they clearly show that the name of Earth was Asia. When the Honorable Elijah Muhammad calls us the "Asiatic Black man" that's "the Maker, the Owner, the Cream of the Planet Earth, God of the Universe," he is saying we are the first man on every part of the 24,896 square miles of this planet. We are the first people to walk on the 57,255,000 square miles of Land. We are the first people to sail the 139,685,000 square miles of water. And yes, we are the first people to travel the 76 quintillion miles of the Universe. We are the Asiatic.

This is why, if you notice no matter where you look, Caucasian people have never claimed to be the native on any portion or part of the Earth. Why, because by definition the word native means to be naturally born or the first born to a specific area. They are not the Native American nor the native Africans. They are not the native Japanese; Chinese not even the native Europeans. When their scholars and their anthropologists, including the Leakey family, excavated for bones to conclusively determine who the Original was, operating from a belief that Aristotle, Plato, Socrates, and Thales were the fathers of art, science and civilization and they were Greeks, they determined that they should beginning digging in Europe. What they found in Europe were the bones of white men and women who were only 6,000 years old; they kept digging. No matter where they dug in Europe, they failed to find any bones of whites older than 6,000 years.

Eventually, they found a set of bones where the measured levels of carbon reduction allowed them to conclude that this particular human being was more than 6,000 years of age. In fact, the testing determined that this set of bones was over one million years of age and the DNA testing determined the genetic structure of the bones to be that of a Black man's bones! Based on these findings, the scientist determined that they needed to take a closer look at Africa; eventually launching a major expedition. During this expedition, they found bones that were 6 million years old, 10 million years old and 50 million years old. When they found the bones of this 50 million year old man and they called him Zinjanthropus; 'Zinj' meaning Black, 'anthropus' meaning human being. Why because the oldest bones they found were those of a Black man. The expedition took place in Egypt where the Great Pyramid of Giza; 451 feet tall, 451 feet deep, covering thirteen and a half acres made of 1 million, three and a half ton blocks of gold and granite stacked mathematically precise, not deviating, not even by a square inch, built without a modern bulldozer or crane. Built by the Black Egyptians, using the power of their mind in a collective manner, which allowed them to mentally renegotiate the stones, in spite of the size, in a perfect mathematical way. Constructing a magnificent architectural and structural wonder that still fascinates to this day.

Resting at the base of this Great Pyramid of Giza, there was a statue that featured the body of a lion with the head of a Black man on it. Many asked the question, 'How do you know that it's a Black man's head on it? Because when you look at it, it seems like erosion has caused the nose and the features to fade away? The tragic reality is that this is not a product of erosion. This is the product of a man named Napoleon, a French military general, who ordered his soldiers to train their cannons (guns) on it to blow off the broad nose and thick lips. Why, because there is something called 'image association.'

The science of image association means that when we see a lion, who is the king of the jungle, and he has the head of a big thick lipped, broad nosed Blackman on it. And if the lion is the king of the jungle and on it is the head of a Blackman, then maybe they are saying to us that we are the king of the planet! Written in Arabic beneath The Sphinx are these words: 'Abu Al Hol', which translates into 'Father of Everything'. The oppressor could not allow an African featured Black face to stay on the body of the lion, because if that image was seen and understood today in a modern context, then it may inspire our young men to pull up their pants and clean up their life. This may inspire our women to wear looser clothing from a desire to cover her hair and body like a queen. This is an image that will inspire dignified behavior causing us to reach up for higher and higher levels of knowledge and not down for alcohol, weed or cigarettes.

A study was done in Harlem, New York, and chronicled by the New York Times in an article written by Mr. Sam Dillian and published originally on January 22, 2009. The article entitled, 'The Obama Effect.' This study reported on what happened when a group of Harlem high school students were tested before Obama became President and 80% of them failed the test. Then, without any additional tutoring, these same students retook the exact same test after Obama became President, and this time around 80% of them passed with exceptional scores. What this study shows is that it was not a case of the Black child not having the knowledge base because they did. He had the knowledge in his head but what was missing was the confidence and motivation needed to bring to the test. This is the reason why it has always been such a struggle, such a hard road, to learn of the true greatness of our real legacy as a people.

When we start school, as a child every child starts school the same way timid, including Caucasian children. When Caucasian children go to school, they learn about Thomas Jefferson and this knowledge raises them up a little bit. They learn about Abraham Lincoln, Thomas Edison, Aristotle and Plato. Which raises them up a little bit. By contrast, when we go to school, we do not learn anything about ourselves. We learn more about our enemy than we do about ourselves. The Honorable Elijah Muhammad described the public school system as a ‘killing field.’ If it is a killing field, the logical question is: What are they killing in our babies when we send them to these schools? The answer is that what they are killing is the spirit of God within in them. They are killing their self-worth, their self-esteem and their self-confidence.

Now, what happens to a Black child’s psyche when he learns more about somebody else than he learns about himself? The Honorable Minister Louis Farrakhan Muhammad teaches us that the knowledge of self produces love for self. Love for self-causes us to do for ourselves. What we know, we love and what we love we do for. And if we do not know our self, then we do not love our self, and if we do not love our self we cannot do right for our self. When we look closely at the word ‘brother’, we can see that the base word of brother is 'other'; our brother is our 'other' self, and he does not stand a chance because it is easy for us to kill one another when we do not know one another.

On a subliminal level, if we learn more about White accomplishments than we do about our own accomplishments then we, on a subconscious level, actually love our enemy more than we love ourselves. Which means we will do more for them than what we will do for ourselves. And this is the reason why when we look at the current dynamic, Black people are the only people on the planet who will blame the White man for 95% of their problems and still spend 97% of our money with them. Something is wrong with that math. Something is wrong, tragically wrong with that math.

We go out to a restaurant or order in and every year; these pizza restaurants have at least one driver putting some extra sauce on the pizzas and it's not tomato sauce; but we keep on ordering from the same place for some reason. Let us go to a Black restaurant, first time they short us one hush puppy. 'See that. See that's why I don't like doing business with these... I ain't never coming back there again. It's supposed to be 16 fries on here, they gave me 14 French fries. I ain't never going back no more.' We hard on one another but we are merciful on our enemy. The scripture says that we are a sheep like people. Easily led in the wrong direction but hard to lead in the right direction. I hope we all realize that there is something very wrong with the sheep because the sheep never attacked the wolf.

Do you realize that there is one dog gathering up all the sheep; two dogs with a hundred sheep? Question: Why didn't it dawn on the sheep, 'Wait a minute, it's 200 of us. I don't want to go that direction.

Look here Lassie, look here Fido, look here Benji, I'm not going that way. Let's turn on them and get what we want.' Well, that's what Black people are like; easily controlled by the wrong and hard to influence with what is right.

The Prototype

Again, what we find in Student Enrollment, Question No. 1, Answer No. 1 regarding the Original man is that God, Himself, is the prototype. When we understand that we are copies of the Original; however, by our sojourn here in the West and what we have been fed in the form of religion, education, diet and the effects of the environment, we have been altered out of our Original state. Therefore, Allah (God) says in the *Holy Qur'an* in Surah 4 verse 3, "*This day have I completed my favor on you, and I have perfected for you your religion. And I have chosen for you Islam as your religion.*" The word 'religion', 're' meaning to do again. 'Ligion' in the Greek means to get to God. So, religion is supposed to be a spiritual process that gets man back to being a god! It is not supposed to produce just a believer, just an apostle, or a disciple or a companion or a worshiper.

No real religion, if it only produces a believer, apostle, disciple, companion, deacon, bishop or worshiper, if this is where it stops at, you and I really do not have a real religion. If all our religion promises us that we will be a good follower and a saint at the end of the process, then we are not in the religion of God. We are in are in a religious system defined and upheld by men for their gain not our gain, growth, or development. If religion, by definition of the word, means to get us back into the oneness with God, then there is absolutely no other religion on Earth, but the Life-Giving Teachings of the Honorable

Elijah Muhammad that teaches that God can be a man and man can be God! This day we have a perfected religion!

There something called acronyms, where each letter represents a different word. For example, FEAR: False Evidence Appearing Real. That is why they say there's nothing to fear but fear itself. Luck, there's no such thing as luck. You can step on as many cracks as you want, break as many mirrors as you can. Hold onto a four-leaf clover or get you a rabbit's foot — I just want us to stop and think here: how can a rabbit's foot bring us good luck? When the rabbit we got it from used to have four before we got that one and he wasn't so lucky with four of them! Naw, this is 'stupidstition'. No, I didn't say 'su', I said 'stupidstition.' There is no such thing as luck in the sense that something just going to happen by some magic. Luck is also an acronym meaning: **L**aboring **U**nder **C**orrect **K**nowledge. When we work to exhaustion and our effort is being guided by correct knowledge then we can call ourselves a lucky human being.

One writer turned the word Islam into an acronym. With Islam meaning: the Ideal System of Living for All of Man. This is an excellent description of what Allah (God) revealed to Prophet Muhammad (PBUH) in the *Holy Qur'an*, which has been explained to us by the Honorable Elijah Muhammad and the Honorable Minister Louis Farrakhan. We learn from the *Bible* that man was created or made in the image and the likeness of God. Meaning, we look like God on the outside, that's image. Likeness, meaning we even look like

God on the inside. The 99 Attributes of Allah (God) are all human characteristics. The difference between Allah (God) and His use of the 99 attributes that He possesses and our use is that, He has absolute mastery over them and knows at what percentage to apply each attribute and in what combination. He knows how to use them in balance and we do not yet possess this knowledge.

What this means is that we are 'The Avenger' when we should have been 'The Merciful.' We are ready to cause death and destruction when its time give mercy and encourage life. We are trying to be the one that retaliates when we should be, at the time, the one that forgives. Allah (God), He knows exactly what to do and when to do it and the exact percentage or level to do it at. He has mastery over all of the Attributes! Well, if God, Himself, is the prototype the next thing we need to do is find out what will be the process to help us achieve absolute restoration back to our Original state.

Our Father...

"The Bible is our road map to salvation when it's properly understood."
—Honorable Minister Louis Farrakhan

The Honorable Minister Louis Farrakhan made a profoundly brilliant and revolutionary statement in one of his many messages. He explained, "The *Bible* is our road map to salvation when it's properly understood." Meaning, that we actually can study, in the right spirit and manner, the Scriptures and find in them, the process by which we can become an exact reflection of the prototype — God Himself. Most of us have turned Scripture, based on this world's teaching into a holy 'history' book. However, the Most Honorable Elijah Muhammad states in Message to the Blackman that the *Bible* is nearly two-thirds (2/3rds) prophecy.

Prophecy, 'pro' meaning advanced and 'phecy' meaning to speak. That means two thirds of the *Bible* was spoken in advance of it actually happening, actually occurring — future events. So even though the *Bible* was written 2,000 or 4,000 years ago, two thirds of what we read, that was written, did not actually take place during the time of its writing. The prophets who knew how to see into the future, who were recorded, wrote, in advance, what was come. The Most Honorable Elijah Muhammad teaches us regarding even the *Holy Qur'an* that two thirds of it is for him and the other third is for another man in the future, stating directly, "I'll let him worry about his part."

The Honorable Elijah Muhammad was not referring to somebody that lived before him. He clearly stated that he would let 'the other fellow' worry about his part. The 'other fellow' at the time of his making this statement then means, that at that moment, he hadn't begun to fulfil his portion one hundred percent at the time. The question then is, who was the other portion of the book actually for? The answer: it is for a Black man born in North America named the Honorable Minister Louis Farrakhan. He is fulfilling that other third of the work of Muhammad.

When we look at these books, these books are not stories of the past. They are stories of the present. In other words if they were not, why refer to it as a 'living' *Bible*? If it's called a 'living' *Bible*, this means what we read exists in present time, the present moment. The *Holy Qur'an* and *Bible* are both called 'Scriptures'. The base word of scripture is 'script.' A script is a pre-recorded document that is written in advance for a play or movie. Long before the stage is set and the cameras have been turned on, writers write a script to tell the actors where to stand, what to say, what to do and most importantly, when to do it. Well, when you see the *Bible* and *Holy Qur'an* as a 'scripture', this means that God wrote this in advance. Not for a movie, not for a play but on the grand stage of human life where we are the actors and actresses that have a role to fulfill. Unfortunately, some of us do not believe this truth.

Have you ever wondered why you never read last names in the *Bible* or the *Holy Qur'an*? There are no last names recorded in either book. You say, 'Well, wait a minute, Jesus Christ.' Christ is not his last name. Christ is his title. Christ means one that comes to crush the wicked in the last days. What's Daniel's last name? What was Moses' last name? What was Abraham's last name? The last names are hidden because it's not just important to know the person; but what we really are more interested in is learning the characteristics 'of' the person. Why? Because if it is a pre-recorded document then we can read and look at someone's life and then look at the way we are living and say, 'wait a minute, I'm looking kind of like Doubting Thomas right now. Whoa, whoa, whoa, hold on a minute I'm looking a little bit like Nebuchadnezzar right now. Let me come on, alter my thinking and my actions and convert on over to look more like Job. Let me look more like Aaron. Let me look more like Joshua. How did they think? How did they act? And when we think and act like them, then we make them alive all over again.

When we look into the *Bible*, we can clearly identify that there is a process and an image, which shows us what the Original man would look like. In Luke 11:1-4, we find the oft repeated and quoted, *'Lord's Prayer.'* We've all said it at some point, "Our Father, who art in heaven…" A sister asked The Honorable Minister Louis Farrakhan one day this profound question, "How will I know a real man when I meet him?" That's a good question, not only for a sister to be able to identify a good man before she plants her love in the wrong place. It's also a good question we should ask as men, to know what we should be to wear the title, 'Real Man.' The Minister answered the sister and said, "a good description of what a man looks like can be found in The Lord's Prayer." This means that within that prayer, if we unpack it, we will find the characteristics, traits, and the ingredients if you will, of what a man that has been returned to their original state, *A Well Made Man* looks like.

First and foremost, the Lord's Prayer starts with, "***Our Father which art in Heaven***." Well, heaven is traditionally considered to be up, correct? Therefore, if this is a good description of a man, this means that as a man, we have to be somebody that our women and our children can look up to. Heaven is up! And if you are gonna be *'Our Father who art in heaven,'* this means that as men we must be someone that our woman and children can look up to. A woman can't look up to a dumb man, a woman can't look up to a broke man, a woman can't look up to a scared man, a lazy man, a weak man, an immoral man, a punctified man!

A woman needs a man that has a level of insight and intelligence that she can use you as her primary soundboard to bounce ideas off. A man that is looked up to can give his queen deeper insight into the subject and the practical steps to bring into existence whatever she bounces off him. She can call him in a time of trouble or crisis and he has scriptural wisdom and factual empirical knowledge on any subject that eases her mind, because her man knows. When she has a problem at work, she can come home and tell her man that 'this man or my boss said so and so and such and such on the job and he touched me like this.' See, a real man doesn't tell his woman when she's been violated on some enemy's job, 'Look honey, we really need the money. You know you just gon' have to take it for a little while.' Naw, a real man goes and kicks down the door and finds out who violated his woman and becomes the arresting officer, prosecutor, the judge, the jury and the executioner on behalf of his woman! That's what real men do!

The prayer goes on to say, "***Hallowed be thy Name***." Hallowed is something that is greatly revered and honored When a person has a good name, that name is a mark or sign of their overall reputation. This means that a person that has a good reputation is said to be one with noble character. What is character? Character is who we are when nobody is looking. Character is one who operates with integrity. Integrity comes from the Latin word Integer meaning *one*. A man with integrity is one. He's the same in private that he is in public. There are many people who are publicly honorable and noble, but in private, they are dishonorable and foul. The Honorable Minister Louis Farrakhan said this about the great value of Character:

Character is the sea on which knowledge floats. Regardless of how much knowledge you have, your ship of knowledge will sink when you lose your character.

One of the great philosophers by the name of Emerson observed when someone was talking right but not living right. He noted, "What you are is so loud I can't hear a word you are saying."

The Most Honorable Elijah Muhammad defined the epitome of what character looks like. He said after being asked the question: “Have you not learned that your word shall be bond regardless of whom or what?” And the answer, “Yes, my word is bond and bond is life and I will give my life before my word shall fail.” See, that's the highest definition of what character looks like because, this means that if I put my word out there, that I'm gon’ be there, I'm gon’ be there! If I said I'm gon’ do it, I'm gonna do it. If I came to help, I'm gonna help. If I came to work, I'm gonna work. Whatever I came for, I'm gonna do just that unless I'm dead because I gave my word that I would.

Let’s take a deeper look at the question though. There's no footnote attached to ‘there.’ It says regardless to whom or what. Well, a whom is any human being on the planet. That means that there is nothing, no one can do that stops me from keeping my word, no matter what any situation or circumstance comes up. No matter who changes, turns, alters, does what they do or no matter what or how the circumstances, change my word shall be bond. Character is our beingness, and it is beingness x doingness, that = havingness. To be truly successful *A Well Made Man* must not only do good but be good.

"***Hallowed be thy Name***." This means that every brother, every man, without exception, we should be someone that the people in our neighborhood, our community our circle of influence, when they think about us, a smile should come to their face. 'That's Bro So and So. They are always picking up the trash. They always looking out for the children. Those brothers are always making sure that our babies get on the bus safe without no pedophile messing with them.' "*Hallowed be thy Name*."

"***Thy Kingdom come, Thy will be done.***" One side of this means that a prototype of man means that a real Original man willingly subordinates their personal goals, for the goals that come from God. The Original man, *A Well Made Man* will put forth more effort in the establishment of the Kingdom of God than his own individual economic legacy. His primary effort is in service of God by servicing and saving the people of God. The balance of that or the other side of this is that *A Well Made Man*, 'thy WILL be done.' *A Well Made Man* has Willpower not wish-power. The will is the faculty of consciousness and especially of deliberate action. The will is the power of control that the mind exercises over its own actions. Meaning, willpower is not just mind over matter, willpower is mind over mind! Willpower allows a man to check his own stinkin' thinkin'. Willpower activates the override mechanism in the brain, that when pain, fatigue, or distractions show up, you can still execute! *A Well Made Man* does not wish, he wills things into existence. *A Well Made Man* does not wait on the spirit to move him he moves the spirit!

Next it says in the Lord's prayer, "***Give us this day our daily bread.***" Now I don't know about you but where I'm from, we had a lot of different synonyms to describe money. For example, we called money, chips, cheese, bank, scrill, cheddar, dough. Bread? Well, hold on now, what does a real man look like? 'Give us this day our daily bread.' Well, the White man does not give daily bread. He gives weekly and bi-weekly bread. So, in order for us to be a real man, we have to do for self! Own our own businesses! Produce our own industry. Manufacture our own products. Buy our own product and sell it. Set our own hours. Make our own retirement fund. Give us this day *our* daily bread.

There is nothing wrong with money brothers; however, there is something wrong with the mindset that we bring to money. Money is a good servant, but it is a horrible master. Jesus, at one point was asked, "Master, how we can be greater helpers?' He said, "If any man be my disciple, he must first deny himself. Pick up your cross and follow me." When Jesus said pick up your cross, he wasn't talking about picking it up from a kiosk in the mall, from a little jewelry store and slapping it around our neck. No that is not the kind of cross that he was talking about. It has a spiritual meaning to it.

To be honest with you it does not even make a lot of sense to wear a cross in memory of the love of Jesus. Just think about this for a second. If the cross was used as the weapon to kill your man. Think of it this way, if my auntie got killed by someone with an AR-15, I am not going to run around with a gold-plated AR-15 on my neck in memory of my auntie. If my mother, was slain with a 9-millimeter, in memory of my momma I will not go out and get a big ole diamond crested 9-millimeter in memory of her. Well, if the weapon used to kill Jesus was a cross why would we want to wear the cross to show how much we loved him? The cross must mean something far greater and deeper than that.

The Honorable Minister Louis Farrakhan teaches us that the cross represents the struggle within human nature; the spiritual and the mental, that is wrestling with the carnal, the material and the physical — the flesh. Jesus said pick up your cross, then you can have both, but they must be proportioned right — balanced. Notice that a cross has a shorter horizontal line and a longer vertical line. The horizontal represents material things — the physical aspects of life and nature. While the vertical portion represents the mental and the spiritual.

There is nothing wrong with working hard to make some chips, but make sure you have more character than chips. There is nothing wrong with having bread as long as you have more belief than bread. There's nothing wrong with getting your finances together long as you get your faith together. There's nothing wrong with trying to get the dollar, just don't ever put the 'dollah' above Allah (God). As long as you keep it in its right and proper place, money is one of the promises of God that will be a good tool of service in the building of His nation, the Kingdom of God. After we acquire money, we have to convert it to wealth. There is a difference between income and wealth. Income is money you earn for your exchange of a good, product or service. Wealth is what you exchange the money for that either keeps its value or increases in value over time. That's your own businesses. That's real estate. The Most Honorable Elijah Muhammad taught us that there were three sciences that were never taught to the slaves. The science of warfare, mating, and business. When you diagnose our community, we suffer the most in these three essential nation-building sciences. If we knew the science of warfare, we wouldn't kill each other over minor offenses and let the enemy off the hook for major offenses. If we knew the science of mating, which is two sided. One side is choosing a mate. The other side is nurturing, cultivating the product of the bond, and parenting. If we knew the science of mating, we wouldn't have a 75% divorce rate. If we knew the science of mating, mothers and fathers would be the primary influence in our children's life and we would nurture them into being the god's they were born to be! According to Dr. Jawanza Kunjufu, the three most influential forces in the 50s was home, school, and church. In the 80s it was peers, television, and school. In 2007 it was peers, music, and television

Today, you have to add social media. Look at the math. The divine and natural position of parents has been hijacked! The *Science of mating*! The other science, we are dealing with making that 'daily bread' as the Most Honorable Elijah Muhammad called it, The Do For Self Program, owning our own businesses. *The science of finance*. If we knew the science of finance, we would not be blaming the white man for 95% of our problems but spending 97% of our money with them. We would not be the leaders in unnecessary spending. What is unnecessary spending? Buying what you don't need, with money that you don't have, from people that you don't like, to impress people that you don't even know! According to the Nielsen report, Black people brought in $1.3 trillion dollars last year, making us out of 226 nations, the eighth richest nation on earth! We've got dollars. We just need some 'sense' to go with the dollars! We need to learn how to use a dollar. Simple system. Out of countless books and finance programs I've studied, there is a universal theme. Live, not within your means, but below your means. 70/10/10/10 rule is minimum. Live off 70% of your income. The three 10% categories: Investment, Savings, and Charity. That's basic. You want to take it to anther level? Cut into the 70% to have more to invest, save, and give in charity. When buying a house, your mortgage should not be more than 28% of your monthly income. Your car payment shouldn't be more than 10%.

Remember, wherever success is, sacrifice once was.

Here are a few key principles and sayings of a Well Made Man:

- *A good man leaves an inheritance to his children's children,* Proverbs 13:22
- *Invest in seven ventures, yes, in eight; you do not know what disaster may come upon the land.* Ecclesiastes 11:2
- *And those of you who die and leave wives behind, should make a bequest in favour of their wives of maintenance for a year without turning (them) out. Then if they themselves go away, there is no blame on you for what they do of lawful deeds concerning themselves. And Allah is Mighty, Wise. Holy Qur'an* 2:240
- Being broke is hard. Building wealth is hard. Choose your hard.
- Can't have a million dollar dream with a minimum wage workers ethic.
- If you woke up broke. You had no business going to sleep.
- I'd rather be tired with money in my pocket then well rested and broke.
- Don't go broke trying to look rich. Respect is earned not bought.
- I have to rewire my brains: Happiness has to be disconnected from spending and reconnected to saving and investing.

Next we read in the Lord's Prayer, "***Forgive us our sins as we forgive,***" wait, wait a minute. Forgive us ours as we forgive others. 'As,' meaning in the same manner? What are we really saying to The Supreme Being, forgive us the way we forgive other people? Now that is rough. Brothers what this really means is that we must settle our differences as a people. We need each other, whether we realize it or not. *Well Made Men* aren't petty! *Well Made Men* don't operate in resentment. Resentment is letting someone use your mind rent-free. Prophet Muhammad said, "Forgiveness sets a prisoner free." Crazy thing is, the prisoner was us! Incarcerated in the prison of toxic emotions. Therefore, forgiveness is not a gift to the wrong doer. It's really a gift we give ourselves.

Paul said that you can tell when a man has gone from death into life because he loves the brotherhood. Prophet Muhammad, (PBUH) said there are three things you need to remain a Muslim. Allah (God), the Messenger and the community. The *Holy Qur'an* enjoins the Muslims to hold fast to the covenant or the rope of Allah (God) altogether and be not disunited. Why should we hold onto the covenant or the rope of Allah (God) altogether and be not disunited? Because all of us were thrown a rope while we were swimming in the sea of sin. Now imagine, if we were in the sea and Muhammad's Ark comes by and we are all trying to get out of the sea of sin. A rope was passed down from Muhammad's Ark and all of us holding onto the rope. We are all pulling, climbing, in unity trying to get out the sea and into the boat. The beauty of holding fast to this rope altogether, is that if your brother starts to slip a little bit, and you have a firm grip, you can hold on a little tighter with one hand; maybe double the rope around your wrist and reach down and get your brothers hand and hold on to them until they get their spot, their strength back. That's the way Believers should treat Believers!

Allow me to give you a very personal example of this very real principle. At one point, I was training for a marathon, 26.2 miles. That's a very, very long run. I think you burn 70 calories just saying 26.2 miles! My running partner and I struck out on a 21-mile training run. When we first met, he had been running longer than I had, so it was an opportunity to pick up some tips from someone who had run longer than me, I respected his knowledge and his experience. Long story short, I'm running, he's showing me different techniques, I'm showing him some of the things I had learned. The little I knew at the time. However, I am a student of 'How to Eat to Live' and I would constantly advise the brother to eat, 'One meal a day.' Assuring him that the marathon could be run eating this way. He was doubtful and frequently said, 'Brother you gonna die! You gotta eat brother.' I stood firm, 'No sir, one meal a day. We can do this on one meal a day.' He's like, 'Brother, you gotta carb load. You need some pasta!' I'm like,' No sir, that's not the Honorable Elijah Muhammad's Teachings. If I can't do it in accordance with 'How to Eat to Live' then it's not supposed to be done. So I'm gonna 'try'.

Every day, from that point forward, it became a little lightweight competition between us because I wanted to prove to him that there is no God but Allah (God) and Muhammad is His Messenger by every mile we ran. So, we get out there on this, 21-mile, run at around the 17th mile I was hurting real bad, legs starting cramping, just hurting. I looked over at him and his back was straight, his stride was good, and he had a real good pace. You know what I said, within myself? I'm a be honest. I said I'm not getting ready to let no cognac dipping, cheeseburger eating, black and mild smoking negro beat me. If he can do it so can I! That's what I said in my head.

I kept running. We got to the end and we both fell out in the grass. Guess what this brother leans over and had the audacity to say to me? He said, 'Brother I got to tell you something brother. I was hurting really bad around that 17th mile marker. 'But I looked over at you and your back was straight, your stride was good, and you had such a good pace. I said if he can do it...' The point is that we borrowed from one another's strength. Had we been out there by ourselves, we both would have given up at the 17th mile. Being in unity, doing the same thing, I am telling you brothers, we can do it if we stay together and we can do it longer and better in unity. Also, I'm pleased to announce that this running partner, his wife, and his son are now all Registered Members of the Nation of Islam!

It is a scientific fact that a Belgian Horse can only pull 8,000 pounds of weight, by himself. When this same horse, is hooked with another horse like it, the two together can pull 25,000 pounds. In unity there is strength! Don't you know that a single goose can only fly at 12 miles per hour alone but when that single goose joins others, these geese form themselves into ranks in a'V flying shape. If the same goose goes off by itself that goose could only could fly at 12 miles per hour, when it's in unity with other geese it can go 65 miles per hour. The scientists have found that by flying in a 'V 'shape, each bird flapping its wings gives the immediate bird behind it an uplift that adds 71% to each of their flying range. Which means that whenever the geese are in unity they can fly faster and farther! Unity!

Allah (God) states in the *Holy Qur'an* that, He created everything, the animals, all of the birds that fly in communities like yourselves. Meaning, we are supposed to see them only as a sign, but we are created to be better than them. If the Belgian horse and the geese can do it, what would happen if Black people made their minds up to be just as united with God and one another as these lower-level creatures, once and for all. One of the great impediments to our unity is grudge holding for past mistakes others have made. *A Well Made Man* must be conscious and cautious but not petty.

The Lord's Prayer goes on to state, "***Lead us not into temptation and deliver us from evil***." What we need to really understand as men, as fathers, is that our children and children in general, children don't do what we say. Children do what we do. Whether we know it or not, there is a direct biological connection between us and our offspring that allows information to be transmitted from one to the other without even having to speak a word. All mothers know this to be true and factual.

A mother can live in Illinois with her ‘grown baby ’living in California, she can pick up the phone and call and as soon as her baby answers the phone, ‘You been on my mind real heavy. Is everything alright? Something’s wrong. ’And your baby breaks down crying. How did she know? There is a bridge between the parent and the child that transmits data one from one to the other. Even though a lot of us, use deceptive intelligence to make excuses and tell ourselves, you know what, my daughter or my son don’t know I did it because they didn’t see me doing it. ’No, the prayer clearly states, lead us not into temptation but deliver us from evil. This means that whatever we want to see coming from our offspring or from others we are trying to influence, we have to be an example of that.

Leading By Example

"Nothing speaks louder than an example."

—Honorable Minister Louis Farrakhan

The Honorable Minister Louis Farrakhan teaches us that nothing speaks louder than an example and the best way to produce change in others is to "LEAD by example." If we make a personal commitment to BE what we want to see, I guarantee we will be a lot better off. These are some of the ingredients that make up the process that will help us get to the prototype. Well, there was one other thing though in the 3 steps wasn't it? Prototype, process and what else? Proof! Proof is present when we know for certain that the process actually worked. The Honorable Minister Louis Farrakhan and the Most Honorable Elijah Muhammad, these are material witnesses, the supreme example that the process works, they are *Well Made Men*. Their existence bears witness to all of us and the world that we can in fact return back to our Original state!

Historically, one thing that usually happens when we read over history, we have a tendency to say what we would have done had we lived back then? 'Had I been back there during the time of Moses, It would have been Moses and Joshua and me. I would have been the 13th disciple. Harriet Tubman would have been there with her shotgun and I'd been right beside her with that 38. Malcolm would have been on one side with a rifle I would have been on the other side with a

Desert Eagle. I would have been with Martin Luther King. 'Is that right?

Well Allah (God), out of His Grace, He has given us an opportunity in the present time to make our word bond because there is a man on scene today, that when you look at him you can see Muhammad. You can see Jesus. You can see Moses. You can see Aaron. You can see Harriet Tubman. You can see Denmark Vesey, Gabriel Prosser, Marcus Garvey and definitely, the Most Honorable Elijah Muhammad. That man I passionately believe is the Honorable Minister Louis Farrakhan!

When we find one man, who is the manifestation of all of these great men, all of them wrapped up in one, then it's time now for us to make our word bond. You say, 'But there's a few things that I've heard that I'm not quite sure of I don't quite fully understand yet. ' Understanding doesn't come before submission. Understanding is the fruit of submission. A person must have some degree of faith. Who can you turn to that can prove what we believe and what we are teaching is false and of no effect? There is nobody, living or dead, that can prove that the Honorable Minister Louis Farrakhan is telling a lie. Have you noticed that all the name calling that the Jews and the media have done, for years? The wicked work of the government that's been done against us, for years. Have you noticed that they called him an "anti-Semite"? They have called him a "bigot, a racist, a hate teacher, homophobic". A "hater". But one thing you **never** heard them call the

Honorable Minister Louis Farrakhan is a liar because they know in their hearts and based on their knowledge of history that the man is telling the truth, they just refuse to publicly admit it.

The Most Honorable Elijah Muhammad challenged the minds and the so-called facts, that you will read designed to turn you against these Divine Teachings during the Theology of Time. During the Theology of Time lecture series, the Most Honorable Elijah Muhammad stated, ***"If you can prove what I teach to be a lie then I will give you one hundred thousand dollars out of my brother's vest pocket."*** Boy that's bold!

When we were growing up we would always say when people started talking, 'put your money where your mouth is'. Well, the Most Honorable Elijah Muhammad said that ***"'what I got, I got from God. I was taught by God. I met with God. I ate with God. I drove with God. I wore God's clothes and I was taught for three and a half years by God in Person. Prove me that I'm a liar. There is a Mother Wheel."***

After he put it out there, not one single person came forward to challenge him. We all know what it means when you really want to prove a point, you up the ante. The Most Honorable Elijah Muhammad came back and stated, ***"I will give any of them $20,000 an hour to come and contend with me."*** That's some bread! Would you agree? None of the scholars, none of the scientists showed up.

None of the learned theologians showed up. The Most Honorable Elijah Muhammad took it even farther. He said, ***"If you can prove what I'm teaching to be a lie, I'll give you $10,000 per word."***

Let's run the math on this. There are 110,500 words in the ***Message to the*** Black man, 83,525 words in ***Fall of America***, 70,850 words in ***Our Saviour Has Arrived. How to Eat to Live Book One*** and ***Book Two*** have 113,750 words combined. If the Honorable Elijah Muhammad was lying, the person who proved him to be a liar would have collected $3,786,250,000.00 (three billion, seven hundred eighty-six million, two-hundred fifty thousand dollars) yet, none of them showed up to challenge the Messenger of Allah (God), the Most Honorable Elijah Muhammad!

My point brothers is that there is no Google search, no library you can go to and find anyone that can defeat the life giving Teachings of the Most Honorable Elijah Muhammad! What he was given by Allah (God) is the process that will get us back to our original state, the living expression of the Lord's Prayer. The best way to prove that we would have been soldiers for the great ones of the past, is by being a soldier for the great one in the present. Not just celebrating and supporting, but becoming *A Well Made Man* like he is.

God is a Man of War

(Exodus 15:3)

If God is a Man of War and in our original form, we are created in His Image and after His likeness, we too should be Men of War. We live in a world that is diametrically opposed to our rise as a people in general, and the Black man's rise in specific! Whatever we are, whatever field we operate in, we have to attach soldier to it. Soldier lawyer, soldier doctor, soldier chemist, soldier banker, soldier teacher, soldier engineer, soldier! In order to thrive or even survive, the Black man must always keep a militant posture and a soldier spirit as we work and live.

Look at the lessons in the training of the men in the Nation called the F.O.I. (The Fruit of Islam). When you enlist into the FOI, you become a soldier in the *Army of Allah* (God). We have one National Song in the Nation, not the prayer song, not the study song, but the Fight Song! The Most Honorable Elijah Muhammad said, "Make all men and boys join the FOI. Train the fast and make them brave fighters, willing at any time to give their lives for Allah's sake and righteousness." Then in the *Holy Qur'an*, Allah says, *"Fighting is enjoined on you, though it is disliked by you; and it may be that you dislike a thing while it is good for you, and it may be that you love a thing while it is evil for you; and Allah knows while you know not. And they will not cease fighting you until they turn you back from your religion."* (*Holy Qur'an* 2:216-217) It seems like Allah (God) is telling us, I know you may not want to fight all the time, but you better gird up your loins and embrace the fact that *A Well Made Man* is a soldier that does not run from the fight, but runs to the fight!

In Islam, one of our prayers says this, "*My prayer, my sacrifice, my life, and my death are all for Allah, the Lord of the worlds.*" Look at the divine order in this prayer. Many people you meet in the world. Enter the mission and in various movements say, "I will die for this!" However, my prayer, sacrifice, life and, death. We wont *die* for what we won't *live* for. We wont *live* for what we wont *sacrifice* for. We wont *sacrifice* for what we wont *pray* for. It starts with our petition to Allah and is followed by our varying degrees of activity after the petition that proves we are sincere and serious. Sacrifice for it. Live for it and die for it when the time arrives. Giving our word to God and each other has to mean something. In fact, Master Fard Muhammad asked the Most Honorable Elijah Muhammad a question that is found in our Supreme Wisdom Lessons. *Have you not learned that your word shall be Bond regardless of whom or what?*

Yes.

My word is Bond and Bond is life, and I will give my life before my word shall fail. "Is" in Mathematics is the same as the equal sign. Whatever is on the right and left of the equal sign has the same power and function of each other. So if "Word = Bond = Life, then the real way we prove sincerity and seriousness is not talking the talk but walking the walk. The answer from the Most Honorable Elijah Muhammad is the true definition of commitment. He's saying, when I put my word out that I'm going to be or do, I will give my life before I fail. This the way we must all be if we are to be *A Well Made Man*. *A Well Made Man* does not quit when he's tired, we quit when we are done!

A *Well-Made Man*, is a soldier, a thinker, a disciplined man, who can handle himself and who is committed to being a Saviour of his people and an example of what 'salvation looks like for our people. And since salvation in Hebrew is Yesha and in Arabic is Khalas, which both mean, to be completely saved, mind, body and soul or spiritually, mentally, and physically (Physical is more than just body. It includes money and all forms of matter. To be completely saved, a man must have his mind, body, soul, and pocket in a healthy and thriving state.) It is in the very nature of a man to not feel complete or *A Well Made Man* unless all these areas are operating on a high level in a man's life. This is why men are magnetized to the example and explanation of the Honorable Minister Louis Farrakhan. He is that completely saved, completely repaired *Well Made Man*. He is the VFP of The NOI. (Valuable Final Product of The Nation of Islam.)

Lothrob Stoddard, a racist historian and journalist writes in his book called *The New World of Islam*, *"Islam is the natural religion of the* Black man *that brings out of the* Black man *his militant propensities."* This is the reason why no other spiritual movement on the planet has young Black men in a respectable number except the Nation of Islam under the leadership of the Honorable Minister Louis Farrakhan. The Black man is demagnetized from any system that does not marry religion with revolution; spirituality and our struggle; faith with the fight and worship with warfare! The F.O.I. are a different breed of spiritual people, Allah in the person of Master Fard Muhammad described the meaning of F.O.I. as ***"The name given to the military training of the men who belong to Islam in North America."*** He purposely attached to our spirituality, the struggle to free our people. He purposely attached our religion to the idea and concept of the revolution. We have one song we sing in the Nation of Islam, "The FIGHT song." Our book, the *Holy Qur'an* has chapters called The Allies, Chapter 33. Those Ranging in Ranks, Chapter 37 The Companies Chapter 39. (That's Military language). This use of military language should indicate to the Black man that the attitude, disposition, and spirit desired by Allah (God) for us, is that of a warrior, soldier and a fighter.

There is no Mystery God! The Most Honorable Elijah Muhammad in his illuminating book, *How to Eat to Live Book 1* on page 58 writes, ***"Remember, life is what we make of it."*** We are not creatures of circumstance; we are creators of circumstance! The *Bible* says in Genesis chapter 1 that man was given power and dominion over the fish of the sea, the foul of the air, and every creeping thing that crawls on the earth. The *Holy Qur'an* in 14th chapter says that

Allah (God) made subservient to man everything in the heavens and the earth and all in between it. This means we are not supposed to sit around and wait on the Spirit to move us. We get up and move the Spirit!

The Honorable Minister Louis Farrakhan lays out the formula of achievement and the recipe of success in any endeavor in a message titled, "Belief in Allah" delivered in 1994.

"When thought germinates in the mind, if you continue to think on the thought, then the thought without more thought only is a thought that comes and goes. And you will say when somebody else comes up with the thought, but thinks on the thought, "They stole my idea!" "They making the money and I ain't got nothing. Low down dirty thief"

Wait a minute fool; you don't have any corner on thought. You don't have any specific corner on imagery. Many of you have good thoughts but you do nothing about what you think. So the thought was an opportunity that you blew, because you didn't do by the thought what you should have done. You've got to think on the thought! You have to think on the thought and thinking on the thought is feeding the thought and then the thought develops into an idea and that idea had with it a plan, a scheme, a method of fulfilling and concretizing what was a mental image that had potential but now you want to actualize what you have envisioned. But if you even develop the thought into a idea and still will not work the idea. Then

God will give the idea to somebody else who will fulfill their idea and fulfill the vision brought by the idea.

Beloved brothers and sisters listen, after the thought brings up a concept, you've conceived. Most people talk the thought and then thought gets lost. It's like showing the baby before the Baby is a baby. Who wants to see a clot but an abortionist? And most times we get a thought, we speak it before we think on the thought. Get it developed and it must develop in darkness. Like the womb of the female, the womb of the mind, develop your ideas, then develop the method, the plan of execution. The idea will bring up a picture of the completed thing. The picture is on your brain. You can draw it on a piece of paper. So that you can keep the vision before your eyes, but putting it on paper isn't actualizing the vision. The vision is only actualized when you bring it into concrete reality. How do you bring it into concrete reality?

First, without faith, you can't work the vision. Even if you see it, you have to now believe that you can bring it. Not only believe in God but believe in yourself! Believe that you can do what you envision that must be done. But belief alone is not of any value unless it is translated into practice or work. And it is belief joined by work that concretizes vision."

In this message the Honorable Minister Louis Farrakhan says, "the first step to the achievement of any goal is to ***"entertain the thought***

free of doubt." Is this why the Most Honorable Elijah Muhammad said thought travels on average at the speed of 24 billion miles per second. Toxic food and toxic thoughts slow down thought. Doubt is a toxic thought. It is entertaining faithlessness in the God and self that will slow down the speed of thought. In physics the formula for Power is Work divided by Time. This means speed is power. Slower moving thought equals a less powerful thought. You and I, having a thought traveling in our brain at an average of 24 billion miles per second, in a circular motion, around 14 billion brain cells, By the law of centrifugal force we repel people, situations and circumstance that are the opposite of our thoughts. By the law of centripetal force, we attract people, situations and circumstance that are in accord with the nature of our thoughts.

Prophet Muhammad (Peace Be Upon Him), reportedly stated that, when Allah (God) has decreed a certain rank for His servant, that they have not achieved by means of their own actions. Then Allah (God) begins to afflict that servant's body, his wealth, his children…until the servant achieves, by their own actions the rank that Allah (God) predetermined for that servant.

In simple terms, Allah (God) already had us picked out to become a god. Now you might not know this, but the Most Honorable Elijah Muhammad teaches us ***"All Muslims are Allah's…"*** The Supreme Being is The Master over us all and He is not just one that has total control over things, He is the Supreme Example. We call him, "Master" Fard Muhammad. When you have a master tape or master document, that master is used as the original, but it is connected to a duplication process that is designed to reproduce other versions of itself - other gods. Not the exact identical twin but so close that it looks very near correct. This Supreme Being, Master Fard Muhammad is the first perfect man among us. The first perfect man!

When the Originator began to revolve in space, making time, He studied Himself and found within Himself His own imperfection. He did not wait for someone to point out His imperfections; He identified His own imperfections through self-study. Knowing that He, as the Self-Originating Allah, would not physically live long enough to correct this imperfection, the Self-Originating Allah put in motion, advance mathematical systems, circumstances, and events designed to happen with exquisite precision. Moving trillions of years down the line of time, ultimately bringing to birth, a perfect version of Himself (the Self-Originating Allah) in the form of another man — Master Fard Muhammad.

We are called out of a sin sick world, into the ranks of the Allah (God) based on a precise mathematical calculation. The same type of calculations that the Self-Originating Allah used to calculate the time needed to perfect His creation. Brothers, allow me to prove my point by using our history as the example. The Self-Originating Allah calculated 66 trillion years ago that someone would need to blow the planet apart thus making Moon. He understood that for these mathematical calculations to work, at the 50,000-year mark in our calendar history, someone had to be born — (Shabazz) that would take his family into the jungles of East Asia, as they now call it Africa. And 6,000 years ago, a scientist by the name of Yacub, had to gather exactly 59,999 followers, adding himself to make 60,000, to graft the Devil from the Original Man. And upon the successful completion of the grafting process; they would have to be taught how to master the Original Man.

The Self-Originating Allah knew that for His calculations to work, Yacub's grafted people would need to kidnap and hold another people in slavery, a specially prepared people by Shabazz, for 400 years. The Self-Originating Allah knew that after all these events occurred, according to His precise mathematical calculations, that Alfonso would need to travel to the Caucus Mountain region to get a woman, clean her up and through her bring to birth one in the year 1877. One who would be taught by his Father, Alfonso, the wisdom of ***all*** the Scientists. The Self-Originating Allah, the Original mathematical human calculator, realized after His self-creation was complete, that it would take, exactly 76 trillion years, to bring perfection from Himself. The Self-Originating Allah calculated from the time of this realization that imperfection would need to be perfected, in order to perfect His universe to make it into an exact representation of what He had in His mind when He self-originated Himself out of triple stage darkness.

What we are looking at is, *Supreme Mathematics* from the *Supreme Being*. The Most Honorable Elijah Muhammad said that Allah went to war with the triple darkness for eons and eons of time to bring Himself, His home planet, and the universe into existence. In a message titled, *"What is Your Role?"* the Honorable Minister Louis Farrakhan highlights the chief characteristics that the Originator needed to create Himself. The Honorable Minister Louis Farrakhan then goes on to explain that the same traits the God needed to master the triple darkness, man needs to conquer our environment and be a real man, a God.

These are the traits:

1. Vision
2. A Warrior Mind / Spirit
3. Patience
4. Hard -Working
5. Wise (Wisdom)
6. Organization

"A mistake is an unintentional departure from what is right; an error is an intentional departure from what we know is right. These errors and mistakes hinder the full growth and development of the person, so, we outgrow the need to seek refuge in our leaders, political and otherwise, but to seek refuge in the "God of men" is the ultimate place of refuge, for, no matter what mistakes or errors were made in the parenting of our children; no matter how our children were neglected and not corrected, when we get to Allah (God) we have reached Him who is perfect; we have reached Him who suffices all needs; we have reached Him who is the end of all excuses that we make for our failures in life, blaming these failures on those who have stewarded our lives and in some way have failed."

—Honorable Minister Louis Farrakhan

The 12 Leadership Traits of A Well Made Man

"Giving and living our lives for Truth: This is The Greatest Act of Service that we can do!"

—Honorable Minister Louis Farrakhan

As men we have the task and responsibility to 'close the gap' between us and our teachers. Closing that Gap between what we see and believe and want we actually achieve. The Most Honorable Elijah Muhammad has many titles that we use to describe him. We say Apostle, Messenger, Messiah, Christ etc. All of these were good and represent phases of development on the upward trajectory to what he has become in the now. One of the titles the Honorable Minister Louis Farrakhan calls him is, *"The Architect of a New Civilization."* To create a new civilization, the first thing you need is a **man**.

The Most Honorable Elijah Muhammad has so much confidence in one man that he said about him. ***"Everywhere you hear him—listen to him. Everywhere you see him—look at him. Everywhere he advise you to go—go. Everywhere he advise you to stay from—stay from... I say continue to hear our Minister Farrakhan."*** There is something about his physiology, his speech, his insight and foresight that makes him the one that is to be modeled by all who want to earn citizenship in the new civilization. The Honorable Minister Louis Farrakhan represents the ideal application of divine life principles in real time. It is his "Love

Level" and if we make his Love Level our Love Level, it will bring to birth in us, the adequate fight, drive and focus necessary to be successful soldier's for God. What we must take from the Honorable Minister Louis Farrakhan's rise into the level of God-ship he manifests, is that as men, we can and we must go back to our drawing boards, go onto that shelf, in the subconscious mind and dig out of ourselves those goals, dreams, and aspirations we had in our mind and dust them off. Whatever that spirit-killing teacher told you, whatever momma and daddy told you couldn't be done. Whatever somebody in the hood told you, you couldn't be achieved, go and dust off the blueprint, bring it back out and in your mind say, *'All I have to do is be what he is, where I am.'* In other words, be a Brother Farrakhan at what we do. A manifestation of unconditional love, unshakable faith, and extraordinary effort, and whatever you want to be, do, or have will be manifest!

In a message delivered to the Youth Leadership in Philadelphia, the Honorable Minister Louis Farrakhan taught 12 unique leadership traits. If we commit to working diligently to incorporate these traits into our personal integrity and operational standards, we will be successful. The Honorable Minister Louis Farrakhan is our example, the best example in everything we do as men. He is impeccable in his manners and in his actions. He acts with integrity and he never surrender's His faith and commitment to the Divine Teachings of the Honorable Elijah Muhammad, no matter the challenge or opposition, internally or externally.

The Honorable Minister Louis Farrakhan exhibits leadership because he operates from and understands that real leadership is much more than giving commands and instructions. *Leadership is the ability to inspire others to strive to raise their standards morally, spiritually, intellectually and in the areas of personal and group productivity.* We can read and study the work of James Allen, learning to identify the *21 Irrefutable Leadership Principles*. We can pick up the *Seven Habits of Highly Effective People* from Steven Covey, *The Laws of Success: 16 Lessons* as taught by Napoleon Hill. *The 25 Wealth Building Secrets* as taught by Kevin Trudeau, The 19 this, The 8 that, the 4 this and the 32 that, *48 Laws of Power*, *33 Strategies of War* but *Revelation always trumps Speculation!* These 12 traits are a superior grade of teaching, because they originate from the highest grade of teacher, Master Fard Muhammad, Allah (God) in person and the Honorable Elijah Muhammad through their perfected representative among us, the Honorable Minister Louis Farrakhan.

The Honorable Minister Louis Farrakhan is not a regular human being. He is a *super natural* human being. Messengers of God are not like regular people in the sense that, what regular people offer in all truth, is nothing more than well-articulated opinions or guesses supported by life experiences. The Most Honorable Elijah Muhammad said, "9/10ths of what you learn in this world is falsehood, including the sciences." So when we study the empirical knowledge of this world, we have to have a search procedure, firewall, and a psychological TSA set up at the door of our brain! With the word of God through His Messengers, we can shut down the security mechanisms of the mind and accept it all. When a messenger of God speaks, there is no falsehood mixed in. There are no opinions inside of it. There are no hypothesis nor is there any guesswork involved. It is 100% Actual Facts. Facts that you can stand on and accurately calculate the trajectory of the future by.

The Honorable Minister Louis Farrakhan compared the knowledge from a Messenger of God and the knowledge of regular scientists (people) to water. The Honorable Minister Louis Farrakhan said just as we have common water; we also have in this world what is known as common knowledge also known as science. Common knowledge is like tap water. It is clear. It is wet. It is called water; however, it has inside of it fluoride, chlorine and other bacterial life forms that have within them a corrupting faculty or corrupting agent, polluting the water that you are looking at and drinking. However, the Word from the Messenger of God is not common knowledge. It is likened unto rainwater. For just as a cloud is formed, the Honorable Minister Louis Farrakhan says, messengers are formed in the same manner. What exactly is a cloud? A cloud is nothing more than the renegotiation of the Earth's waters.

The Saviour, Master Fard Muhammad teaches us that the Sun and the Moon have a magnetic appeal on the Earth's water.

Drawing on or pulling on the Earth's water, drawing up the water in a mist that the "naked eye can hardly detect." When that mist becomes heavier than the gravitational pull of the Earth, gathering at the ceiling of gravity, which is six miles high, we call that object, a cloud. When that cloud begins to become too heavy for gravity, it distills back to the Earth in the form of rainwater. When the Moon pulls on the water, it pulls or draws it up in an impure state; that water is dirty water. The higher the water rises up into the sky, the more Sun light the dirty water receives and the light of the Sun serves as a purifier of the Earth's water. Therefore, when the rainwater distills back down, it is not like the lake or ocean water that went up. The lake or ocean water that went up was dirty. The rainwater, when it distills back to the Earth, is purified lake or ocean water. When the purified rainwater comes, it causes growth and development better than regular (or common) water can. This is why no matter how long you run your sprinkler in the yard or garden, nothing matches real live rainwater in the stimulation of growth and health in the yard or garden. You can put the sprinkler out there and have the hose on for a whole day, come back the next day and measure maybe a centimeter's growth, but let it rain for 20 or 30 minutes and 20 or 30 minutes can outdo 8 hours of tap water. These exact same principles apply to the teachings of a Messenger of God.

A Messenger of God comes from the dirty polluted water of the people, meaning he has experienced the same trials and tribulations as the people he is placed over. As the Messenger is being pulled up in the atmosphere, the Light of Allah (God) begins to purify them. When they speak knowledge, it's not tap water. It's not common water. It's not regular science. It's Revelation. It's purified water. When we hear from a servant or a Messenger of God, we are hearing not theory, not opinion, not hypothesis, not guess, no, not even traditional science, but what we are hearing is Revelation from the Lord of the Worlds. It is the purest form of knowledge that anybody could ever consume and just like rainwater, it causes our minds to develop and evolve around the word of Allah (God) in a rapid fashion.

Brothers, the point here is that we must be leaders but not leaders as defined by this world's standards. The leadership traits that we want to come to see and understand come directly from the Mind of God through a Messenger of God. The Honorable Elijah Muhammad spoke concerning the Honorable Minister Louis Farrakhan specifically, He said to us all, *"Everywhere you see him, look at him."* This means there has to be something about the way that he carries himself that is the perfect example of how all humans should carry themselves.

The Honorable Elijah Muhammad also said, "*Everywhere you hear him, listen to him.*" Why, because to hear and to listen are two different things. To hear means that you interpret sound but to listen means that you not only interpret sound, you define what you have interpreted, and you began to listen not with the two ears but with the third ear, which is a spiritual ear. As we have the two eyes, we have a third ear called the mind; and when we listen with the third ear, we don't just hear the distribution of words, but we learn the meaning of the words and then we begin to communicate like the one we are listening to. This means if he wants us to listen to him there is something about the way he communicates that is the developed model of how we as men, should communicate. Then the Honorable Elijah Muhammad said, "*Everywhere he advise you to go, go*" and "*Everywhere he advise you to stay from, stay from.*"

The Honorable Minister Louis Farrakhan is qualified to *inspire* and to *instruct*. The Honorable Minister Louis Farrakhan is qualified to explain everything to us and if we are to see him, not just to look at but also, to see him through the third eye, then he is qualified to be an example for us. To *see* means he is ***the example***. *Hear* means that he is qualified to be listened to; to be guided by, instructed, and inspired by. What the Most Honorable Elijah Muhammad is commanding us to do, is to ***study*** this one man that Allah made for us and He doesn't want us just to learn about him, He wants us to learn ***of*** him. Why? Because to learn *about* a man and learn *of* a man are two different types of learning. "Take my yoke upon you, and learn *of* me." (Matthew 11:29)

'The Honorable Elijah Muhammad taught us that Master Fard Muhammad studied 42 years to deliver us...He studied 42 years to deliver us. He was God but He had to study. He was God, He had that potential, but He had to grow into that potential through study. And so the picture you see of Master Fard Muhammad, you see Him reading a book. Because the only way you can save the people is if you know the wisdom that is found, not just in the newspaper or some book that you were trained in in college, but you must know the wisdom in the book that is designed for the salvation of the Blackman. Do you understand? Christ, the Saviour.

Well, if the Honorable Elijah Muhammad, who was among us, laying a foundation for us to work today, has now left our midst but deposited in us his word and the same course of study that Master Fard Muhammad gave him, then why should we study'? It is because you must study to save and deliver the people. On Saviour's Day 1981, I said, and I am quoting now, "It is written in the scriptures, 'I will send Saviours, plural, after them.' "I will send Saviours, plural, after them. Who is the "I?" The "I" who is doing the sending is the one who is the Christ. He says He raises up disciples and He sends them. He is raised, and then He becomes a sender of Saviours. That's heavy, brother. A Saviour. A Saviour. Pick up your dictionary and look up the word Saviour - one who saves. And when you look in the mirror at yourself, look at yourself good, and say to yourself, "I am sent as a Saviour of my black brothers and sisters. I am a Saviour. I am a Deliverer. I am a Redeemer."

Think about those words. You and I are acting under the Saving Grace and Power of the Saviour - The Most Honorable Elijah Muhammad who is acting under the power of the Lord of the Worlds. So we got power to save. How do you know we got power? Because the word of God coming through me saved you. And the word of God coming through you will save anybody who will listen to you if you will study and qualify yourself for your work as a Saviour of our people."

—Honorable Minister Louis Farrakhan

12 Leadership Traits of A Well Made Man (UNPACKED)

"Love is the power. Love is the force. Love is the gasoline or the fuel that allows one, such as myself, to do what I do..."

—Honorable Minister Louis Farrakhan

Brothers there is a difference between learning *of* a man and learning *about* a man. To learn *about* means you learn: that the Honorable Minister Louis Farrakhan was born in New York in 1933, played the violin starting at the age of so and so, etc. That is learning *about* the man. To learn *of* is to look past biography and look into the *biology* that makes the man who and what he is.

The Honorable Minister Louis Farrakhan in *Closing the Gap: The Inner Views of the Honorable Minister Louis Farrakhan,* which in my humble opinion is an exceptional reference book to learn *of* the Honorable Minister Louis Farrakhan; not *about* but to learn *of* him. He says that Jesus told the world or told man to *'take my yolk upon you and learn of me for I am meek and lowly of heart and ye shall find rest unto your soul.'* The Honorable Minister Louis Farrakhan goes on to explain this statement by informing us that, *"Learning of a man is learning the inner workings of his mind which then gives you the spirit out of which he does what he does and this is why God is using him. If you want God to use you..."* The Honorable Minister Louis Farrakhan continues by stating that if you want God to use you, don't just be an *imitation* of his word or his dress, His external manner; but get in tune with His spirit, for then you will become magnetic. In becoming magnetic, you will draw people unto you that you may bring them to him, that he may bring them to the Messenger and that the Messenger may bring them to Allah (God).

The *Holy Qur'an* gives instructions to the Messenger and the Believers. It says to the Believers, *"And be a messenger unto the people as the Messenger is a messenger of Allah to you."* Brothers, what we have the responsibility of, is to try to be to the people what the Messenger is to us. This means our expressed goal must be daily, to strive to get into the inner workings of the mind of the man that is the Messianic man of the moment, who is without question the magnetic one. We can learn *of* him and become magnetic in our attraction in order to run what they call in football a "flea flicker" play. A flea flicker is when the person that gets the ball does not run it but he passes it to another who in turn passes it to another until the team gets the touchdown.

When we look deeply into the Honorable Minister Louis Farrakhan, we find that he consistently exhibits *12 Divine Leadership Traits* that do not come from the *notes* of the Honorable Minister Louis Farrakhan. These traits came from his *mind.* Without using any prepared notes before him; which means, if he was not reading from a piece of paper in front of him, he was taking these traits from the Official Paper called his own brain cells. From his own mind. When he describes the *12 Divine Leadership Traits*, he is not looking out into the world at any CEO or CFO or

Economic Guru or General so and so. The Honorable Minister Louis Farrakhan was looking at his own characteristics, giving us the inner workings of *his* mind to show us how to be as he is.

Trait Number 1: *You must Love to Lead*

The number one trait that the Honorable Minister Louis Farrakhan said that we must have if we are going to be a good leader is the understanding that, leadership is much more about influence than it is about instruction. Because a person has a post or a position that gives them the authority to instruct only, but another person may have no post or position but because of their love, their spirit and their intelligence, they have influence. The one with influence can be a better leader than the one that instructs because the one that has influence is not making or forcing anyone by way of the position to do anything. The one with influence is operating in such a way that they pique the interest in other people where other people want to do (personally desire) what that other person is doing and to be like that person is, so they are asking, how did you become you?

Every single person is a leader on some level, for all of us have influence over not some person, but some group of people. According to the scientists of this world, the average individual has a sphere of influence of 12 people. Through research, they found that those who are adults, their sphere of influence normally is around 50 people. So each one of us has between 12 and 50 people, not necessarily, that we can instruct, but that we do have influence over. Therefore, leadership has to be seen as a job that all of us are operating in; not something that we get whenever we are given stripes and bars and titles etcetera. The number one trait of a leader from out of the mind of the Honorable Minister Louis Farrakhan, is: ***You must love, to lead.*** Not love TO lead but you must love '*comma*' to lead.

Commas are very important. Love 'comma 'to lead, meaning that you have to have love in order to lead, not that you love telling people what to do. The Honorable Minister Louis Farrakhan says in *Closing the Gap*, as he's being questioned by Brother Jabril Muhammad, Bro. Jabril asks him;

"Brother Minister, it is a fact that any of us who had the privilege of working with you up close well knows; anyone who has observed you from a distance, but has a knowledge of you will bear witness to the same. I am referring to your stupendous and the strenuous nature of your travels; which you have kept on a non-stop, going on twenty-two years, in fulfillment of your assignment. It is a fact that you have a schedule which is practically unbelievable, especially the traveling schedule, which is "unreal." To what degree do you feel love motivates and fuels you to do what you do in the way that you do it?"

The Honorable Minister Louis Farrakhan responds to this question by stating,

"That is the answer. Love is the power. Love is the force. Love is the gasoline or the fuel that allows one, such as myself, to do what I do and appear indefatigable, untired, not worn by what one does, and it is precisely because I love so much of what I am doing. I love to impart knowledge. I love to see the eyes of a human being come open to truths that mean something or can be a motivating factor to make their personal lives more meaningful. This is what gives meaning to my own life. As I give, I get; as I feed, I am fed; as I energize others, I too, am energized because I believe that is what I am born into this world to do."

What the Honorable Minister Louis Farrakhan is teaching us is that the love of what you're doing is the primary characteristic of leadership. The Honorable Minister Louis Farrakhan went on to say that *'you can't just love what you do, you have to love who you are doing it for.'* He said and because *'I don't just love teaching and preaching, but I love who I am doing it for 'the 'who 'I'm doing it for is one factor above me but another factor beneath me. The 'who 'I am doing it for beneath me is my people. But the 'Who ' I am doing it for above me is God and His Christ, the Honorable Elijah Muhammad. So because I love teaching and I love the God and the Christ and I love my people, I get life when I give life. I get energy when I give energy."* The Honorable Minister Louis Farrakhan goes on to say, *"Jesus told us that I have given unto you two commandments and on these two hang all the laws and all the prophets."* Number one: "Love God with all your heart, mind, soul and strength." And number two: "Love your neighbor or your brother or sister as you love yourself."

The Honorable Minister Louis Farrakhan goes into deeper detail on this particular trait stating, *"So there are three objects that you must love if you want to lead."* Number one: You've got to love God. Number two: You have to love yourself. If you don't love yourself, you do not love God. How can you love the Creator and hate self which is the product of the creator, the creation? How can you say that you're in the image and the likeness of God and hate yourself but love who you are a replica of? If you love God and you are created in His image and after His likeness, you are His replica, then you are obligated to love yourself because you are a mirror reflection, physically and spiritually of God. Then number three: In order to lead, you must love your brother and your sister. So the number one trait of leadership is we have to love Allah, God, love self.

Does that mean we are not going to be dissatisfied with ourselves? No, if you're not dissatisfied with yourself you might as well jump off the planet because dissatisfaction is the only thing that brings about a change. If we are not dissatisfied, we will never change and if we do not change, we will not grow. We will always have some degree of dissatisfaction, disappointment and frustration. For disappointment, dissatisfaction and frustration are nothing more than an emotional feeling that comes from observing the gap between reality and expectation. When you look at what you know you could be versus what you and I are and then we look in between the reality and the expectation, not of somebody else but of our own selves, then by observing that gap, depending on how big it is, this will determine how dissatisfied we are; how frustrated we are; how disappointed with self we are. The real test is after we observe the gap and get dissatisfied, do we get sad and depressed and lay down and quit? Or do we get up and go to work to try to close the gap, not just between us and the Honorable Minister Louis Farrakhan, us and God, but close the gap between the reality of self and the expected version of self.

Whenever a man is constantly observing that gap between expectation and reality, they don't need a lieutenant, a captain, a minister, a counselor, trainer or life coach. Why? Because you are and you stay self-motivated. You begin to coach yourself. You check yourself. You operate like a military general over your own thoughts, deeds and actions. Looking constantly, measuring the distance from my current reality to my expected version of self. So love of self means, that I have factored in that I'm not necessarily pleased with who I am, but I'm pleased with who I'm becoming. Love of God, love of self, love of your brother and sister, love of what you're doing and love of who we're doing it for. If we love Allah, the Christ, the Honorable Minister Louis Farrakhan and we love our people, that's who we do it for. If we love whatever we are doing to make a contribution to the establishment of the Kingdom of Islam and we love self, we have the first trait.

Trait Number 2: *Belief in Allah (God)*

The Honorable Minister Louis Farrakhan says, *"In order to lead you must believe in Allah."* We cannot be a leader if we do not believe in Allah (God). Unless we understand that there is a power backing us up that when we think about toe-to-toe combat with our open enemy, it appears on the surface that we are fighting a losing battle. Here we are, we don't carry weapons and even if somebody does have one, it was made by the enemy. You say, *'Well you know I got, I got some of them new tools. I got a Desert Eagle. I got a SK. I got an AK.* 'Scratch off the label and see where it was made--in Israel. Go and look at the bullet case and see where the bullets were made; in America. What happens when you finish shooting out the entire round of bullets? You can't call a time out and ask the White man to sell you some more bullets so you can continue to fight the battle. No, when we begin to compare military weaponry, the fact that our open enemy has an ethnic bomb, that they can drop a bomb, filled with a gas into a city that will only kill Black people. White people and others will be able to walk freely but it's designed to kill only Black people. Then when you look at what we are fighting and who we are fighting and how great they are, it looks like we're fighting a losing battle.

We look up and we see the enemy with drones. We look up and we see stealth bombers, B-52 Bomber Planes. They have some jet planes now that can travel faster than the speed of sound. They have a plane that can travel beyond 1,120 feet per second which means you might hear it but you will never even see it! And if you don't believe in a God, you will quit on the battle. But whenever you start thinking about the Mother Wheel, then the B-52 and the stealth don't seem to be too powerful no more! When you start thinking about the bombs on the Bomber Baby Planes then ethnic gas don't look to be so powerful no more! When you learn that there's a God on your side that can speak 16 languages. That this same God has extracted the language of the people on Mars, He can communicate with the birds, controls rain, hail, snow and earthquakes. When you start to think that you've got a God on your team that can make men's minds to think and do as He pleases, then your enemy don't look so powerful no more, because you believe in a God bigger than the White man.

When you are in this kind of work, the resurrection of the dead, trying to do something good for your people, you got to do what you do to please Allah (God), not to please the people. You have to do what you do to get the appropriate response from your Lord, not the appropriate response from the people you are talking to; because the people will always let you down, but Allah (God) will never let you down. The Nation of Islam is not a 'Black Thang. ' The Nation of Islam is a 'God Thang. 'We do not do what we do for our people simply because they are Black. We do what we do for our people because it is the Will of God that Black people be taught, that Black people be purified, that Black people be given the wisdom of the Book and the *Holy Qur'an*. This is the Will of

God. We don't do what we do and then quit if Black people don't respond. We do what we do because it's the Will of God. If we go out with *The Final Call Newspaper* and don't nobody buy it, Allah is God. We are soldiering to please Him, not to please Brother A or Sister B. The Most Honorable Elijah Muhammad said, *"All you can do is give them the Word, but it is Allah Who makes them understand."* It's our job to give the Word.

Trait Number 3: *Always 'We 'Never 'I'*

The Honorable Minister Louis Farrakhan teaches us that, *"In leadership, it's always we, it's never I."* The worst thing that we can ever say when we talk to other people, is *'I '*or *'you.'* The best thing we could ever say when we are talking to people is *'we '*and *'us.'* The minute that we are talking to somebody and we becomes *'I'* or *'you,'* we have immediately cut the invisible bridge between your mind and the mind of the one to whom we are speaking to, because *'I'* means I'm separate from you and *'you'* means you're separate from me. So *'you'* need to, *'you'* need to do, why because *'I'* already have. When we say *'we'* and *'us',* we recognize that we are all on the same team trying to get help. In fact, any of us that would be asked a question or interviewed and if somebody asked us are you greater than Jesus, all of us would shake our head and say no. But as great as Jesus is he said that "I can of my own self do nothing." Well, if Jesus needs help then all of us need help. There is no such thing as one person doing it all. *'I'* is the only independent letter in the alphabet and it's reserved for the only One that is Independent. The *Holy Qur'an* puts it this way, "Say He, Allah, is One. He Begets not nor is He Begotten. He is the one on whom we all depend." Right? But Allah is Independent. If Allah is the only independent, upon Whom we all depend, then He's the only One that can justifiably say *'I'*. All the rest of us must say 'we'.

Look at Moses, are we greater than him? No we must shake our head and say No sir. Moses, out in the wilderness one day, Children of Israel complaining and Moses came with his stick and said, *"Must I smite the rock and bring forth water?"* He smote the rock, water came forth. But Allah (God) came down from Heaven and said, in so many words, 'Who do you think you are? 'And as a result of Moses using *'I'* instead of saying, *'Must I smite the rock in the Name of Allah'* or *'Must I petition Allah to bring forth water from the rock when I smite it.* 'Because he did not put the *'Inshallah'* on it, *'If it be the Will of Allah'* and he took the authority to say *'I'*. He lost the Promise Land dying before the Children of Israel entered into it. If Allah would do Moses like that and we're not greater than him, we must be careful not to use '*I*', because it's always *'we'*.

Trait Number 4: *Be Nonjudgmental*

The Honorable Minister Louis Farrakhan says, *"We must be nonjudgmental."* What does it mean to be judgmental? To be judgmental means to make a moral judgment. Which does not mean that we walk around stupid and let anything go, *'I mean, Allah's gon judge em.'* No, you have the obligation to protect the community. It is reported that Prophet Muhammad, (PBUH), said "*That no one in the community is held accountable for the wrong of another until they know the wrong of the other and do not report it to those who can fix it.*" The minute that we know of what someone is doing in the community that is wrong and we do not do something about it, we inherit the consequences that the wrongdoer would get. *'They stole a thousand dollars.'* You know it, you don't get a dime of the money but you don't report this crime. Since you knew it, didn't tell, you didn't get any of the money but you get the punishment. What the Honorable Minister Louis Farrakhan is saying to us is that we don't make a moral judgment of condemnation of a person. No matter how grave an offense might be, none of us are qualified to judge another. The Scripture says, 'where there is life there is hope. 'As long as Allah (God), Who takes souls by night, has decided to return a brother or a sister's soul that they can wake up in the morning; which means that by the fact that they woke up in the morning; that Allah (God) still believes in them. In their ability to achieve the rank that He predetermined for them before they were even in their mother's womb. If God believes in them, who are we to disbelieve?

To be judgmental means that we condemn a person forever for a mistake that they have made. Prophet Muhammad (PBUH) said that whenever your brother or sister does wrong make 70 excuses for them. Seventy, before you condemn them. Jesus took it to another level though. Peter came to him in Matthew 18:21 and said, *'Lord'* (he's complaining), *'Lord you mean that we should forgive our brother or our sister seven times for sinning against us?'* He says, *'No, not seven, seven times seventy.'* Four hundred and ninety times; they don't even talk about it no more after that. How do we know, because in the next verse, it goes on to a whole new subject, Peter was like, 'Forget it, I ain't gon talk about this no more. Four hundred and ninety times!'

Trait Number 5: *Service to Others*

The Honorable Minister Louis Farrakhan said that a leader must be the chief servant. "Jesus said I came not into the world to be served, but I came to serve others". Do you know that every time the Honorable Minister Louis Farrakhan comes to answer the phone, when he gets on the phone, listen to his words: *"As-Salaam Alaikum, how may I serve you?"* every single time he gets on the phone. *'How may I serve you.'* Damon Dash posted a picture on Instagram at one point where he was at the farm in Michigan with the Honorable Minister Louis Farrakhan. The Honorable Minister Louis Farrakhan was taking him on a tour, showing Mr. Dash the greenhouse. In one of the photos taken, the Honorable Minister Louis Farrakhan is in his golf cart, Damon Dash is sitting in the passenger seat and the Honorable Minister Louis Farrakhan is driving the cart. The Honorable Minister Louis Farrakhan is not only the honorable but he's also the humble. He didn't have somebody driving them around. *He* was driving *his* guest. Chief servant!

Whenever we seek leadership brothers, we should never seek leadership with the goal of looking for a post to get some privileges, but we should want a post so that we can have a platform that we can perform better than what we are performing at currently, at a higher level, wherever we are located.

Number 6: *You Must Be Humble*

The Honorable Minister Louis Farrakhan says to be a leader, *"You must be humble."* On page 68, of *Closing the Gap,* Brother Jabril Muhammad states,

"This is a two part question. Would you say that your wonderful sense of humor has been a factor in your ability to persevere under the most difficult set of circumstances? And what are some of the other factors that have enabled you to so persevere?"

The Honorable Minister Louis Farrakhan responds,

"Yes, and I also think the greatest factor in my being able to persevere is being blessed to be humble enough to see the Greatness of Allah (God). I know that I am just an atom in the universe of billions and trillions ad quadrillions of atoms. I know that I am so blessed to be able to serve Allah (God), in this time, and in this way. In serving Allah (God), our people and humanity as best I can, and not taking myself seriously in terms of who I am and how people view me, I think, is the underpinning of my sense of humor. This is the underpinning of longevity and perseverance. This is the reason the evil that people do to me really does not affect me; it is because they never reach me. They cannot find me. I am so low to the ground that everything they shoot at me always goes above me; and they could only hit me if I began to think more of myself than I should."

Understand what the Honorable Minister Louis Farrakhan is saying here. In the science of warfare, as soon as you hear a gunshot, what do they say? *'Get low.'* Spiritually, this means get humble and as long as we stay low or stay humble, then we will not be a victim of any of the enemy's attacks. In the *Self-Improvement the Basis for Community Development Study Guides*, Official Edition, the Honorable Minister Louis Farrakhan states,

"At the core of his thinking, the humble man does not think grand things of himself that exalt him above others. It is not a feeling that he is undeserving but is a quality that a leader must have to lift up the weight of the people. The power of strength is in place and it's underweight. The leader cannot pull people from above; the leader must get under and lift them up."

Notice that the Honorable Minister Louis Farrakhan explains that it does not mean that you feel undeserving. True humility does not come from looking down on yourself. True humility comes when you're looking up to Allah (God) and no matter how great you are you see Him as so Great that your greatness is nothingness in the sight of Allah's Greatness.

Number 7: *Honesty, because liars cannot lead*

"A leader has to be honest." The Honorable Minister Louis Farrakhan says, *"Liars cannot be leaders."* We must to tell the truth. Our *Supreme Wisdom Lessons* instruct us to "Speak the truth

regardless to circumstances or events." In the truth is our power, our integrity our connection to Allah (God).

Number 8: *Acquire Knowledge*

"A leader must have knowledge." If we are going to be above people, we have to be above people. If we are going to be in front of people, we should be in front of the people; in multiple areas but definitely in knowledge. What we find in the study of leadership is that ability and effectiveness are two different realities. Ability will always be greater than effectiveness. If a person's effectiveness is a 5 their ability is a 7. The only way to increase their effectiveness in leadership up to 7 is that they must raise their leadership up to 9. Effectiveness will always be a couple of notches below ability or knowledge. The Honorable Minister Louis Farrakhan goes on to say,

"Therefore in leadership one must study to improve themselves, study leadership in and of itself but not study so much that we don't soldier. Remember the Supreme Wisdom says that this title of 'god 'can be accomplished with very little study."

The recommendation is that we study 1 hour a day. Not 3, 4, 5 hours a day of study. What good is it for us to study 4 or 5 hours a day and have no converts? Studying, but no soldiering. Its 'better to soldier and study a little than to study a lot and soldier a little. This goes for business, health, and every category of life. *We cannot win the game in the huddle!* This is what studying is. Studying is huddling. At a certain point, you gotta go and run the play. Huddles are short, the game is long. Studying gotta be short. Working what you've studied gotta be long.

Number 9: *High Morals*

"A leader must have high morals." Morals are defined as, "a person's standards of behavior or beliefs concerning what is and is not acceptable for them to do." This means that we cannot just sway with the wind. Bowing down to anything and everything that comes our way. We must maintain a standard. When our women and children see us, they must know who we are not just by our words, deeds and actions, they must know us by our look — *our very presence should speak to them.* The bulk of all communication is non-verbal. Meaning, you say more with how you look, by your presence, than what you actually speak out of your mouth. Do we look like the Men who belong to Muhammad? What does your presence say? We can't be a *real men* with sagging paints and skinny jeans on. We can't be real men dirty and unkempt, with a mouth filled with slang and cuss words. No! Muhammad makes Men! Our carriage, our posture, our atmosphere we carry us the product of our morals. Having high moral standards means, we don't get reports of you at the strip club. Your wife is not reporting you for beating her or taking off your daughters. Bounty hunters not staking out the Mosque looking for you because you got a warrant out for your arrest. Real men with high morals and standards are not a masculine copy of a gossiping girl. No backbiting, no slandering, no gossiping, no seed dropping, no

hatin', no excuse making, no complaining. Believers train and Hypocrites complain!

Number 10: *Leaders Don't Complain*

"Leaders", the Honorable Minister Louis Farrakhan states, *"Do not complain."* Leaders do not complain. "Have you not learned that your Word shall be Bond regardless to whom or what?" The answer is: "Yes my Word is Bond and my Bond is Life and I shall give my life before my word shall fail.' "Whom 'is anybody on the planet and 'what 'is any situation or circumstance. There is no person nor predicament that I can ever blame for anything, why, because leaders don't complain. Our Ninth (9th), General Order, is what? "To allow no one to commit a nuisance on or near my post." When you unpack these two statements, "Word shall be bond regardless to *whom or what* and allow *no one* to commit a nuisance... They inform us that we are not creatures of circumstance, we are creators of circumstance. We are not effect, we are cause. A leader can never blame anyone or complain about anything. We, as leaders, as men, have to take full responsible.

Number 11: *Cultivate Growth in Others*

The Most Honorable Elijah Muhammad said, "No one man can ever ride above the condition of his people." "We will all be one or nothing." The Most Honorable Elijah Muhammad told the Minister as he was showing the Minister the National House (the home built by the Most Honorable Elijah Muhammad). The Most Honorable Elijah Muhammad told the Minister, Muhammad will not be in this fine home with his feet in the air. Muhammad will be in this home strategizing on how he can put all of the 22 million in one just like it! A real l*eader works to see others grow not just themselves."* This "I got to get mine, you get to get yours. Every man for himself" is a Eurocentric concept we've adopted from the white man. Before we were kidnapped and Caucasianized and Westernized we lived by these African Proverbs: Cross the river in a crowd and the crocodile won't eat you. Many hands make light work. In Islam we are given this principle by Allah (God) through Prophet Muhammad (PBUH) "you are not a Muslim or a righteous person until you love for your brother that which you love for yourself." The Honorable Minister Louis Farrakhan states, *"True leaders want others to value the service, grow from the service and become what you are leading them to and then do for someone else what you did for them."* He sets the example. He knows the way and shows the way. When you're following a leader you should eventually transform to become like the leader you are following and you prove that you're like he is by doing for somebody else what he did for you.

Number 12: *Health*

"A leader must have good health," must be in good health. Every letter that the Honorable Minister Louis Farrakhan writes to anyone, he always opens it in the same way, *'May this correspondence find you in the best of health and spirit.'* These must be the two most important things in life: health and spirit. The synergism of these two things operating at the same time in one

organism makes the possessor an unstoppable man! The Honorable Minister Louis Farrakhan goes on to explain, *"The body has to be kept in a certain way in order for it to be worthy to carry the spirit of life."* This means Allah (God) chooses, He discriminates, He determines the body He wants to live in and if we don't take care of the body Allah (God) can choose, The God might say, *'I'm not giving that much of Me to that. I don't want to live there. Too many Pork chops, Flaming Hot Cheetos in there. I don't 'want to live in there, next to all them Ramen Noodles. I'm not posting up next to no ham sandwich. I wanna live in a body that's a house (a body) that's clean, that's stable, and strong. '* Allah (God) has the right to select and be selective on where He wants to operate, dwell, and reside. Our body, but God's temple!

The Honorable Minister Louis Farrakhan goes on to state unequivocally that, *"Sickness is not natural."* The question is what is natural? *"Health is natural...When we are sick, something is wrong with the way we* ***think****, the way we* ***live*** *or what we are* ***eating*** *and* ***drinking****."* We want to be healthy and fit. *Fitness* and *health* are not the same thing. *Fitness* is the physical ability to perform an athletic action, while *health* is the state of being where all of the systems of the body are working in an optimal way. To be a maintainer, protector, provider, combat ready, it's not 'either or' it's 'both and.'

The Honorable Minister Louis Farrakhan explains that good health means that we, *"Exercise to ward off the force of gravity."*

This is a divine instruction. Exercise, the Honorable Minister Louis Farrakhan's recommendation is that we exercise at a minimum of 30 minutes per day. He says, *"The only way that the Earth doesn't pull you back in, is you must have sufficient energy to ward off the force of gravity. In order to ward off the force of gravity you must eat the right foods and do some exercise."*

These are *12 Divine Leadership Traits* of a leader from the mind of God's man, the Honorable Minister Louis Farrakhan. A trait is defined in one dictionary as a "distinguishing quality (as of personal character)"; it is also defined as an "inherited characteristic." To inherit means, "To receive as one's portion; come into possession of." It also means to "receive qualities, powers, duties, etc. as by inheritance." When we practice these *12 Divine Leadership Traits,* as defined and exemplified by the Honorable Minister Louis Farrakhan, striving to follow his example perfectly, wherever we are, we will become magnetic in the same manner that he is magnetic.

We will draw people unto us and when the people are attracted to us, we will not seek to satisfy our egos out of vanity and keep the people tied to us. All of us will have become the kind of leaders that the Honorable Minister Louis Farrakhan is. We will have studied him so deeply, that we will have learned **'of'** him and have become **'of'** him.

Well Made Man Leadership Traits Summary

1. *Love to Lead*
2. *Belief in Allah (God)*
3. *Always 'We 'Never 'I'*
4. *Be Nonjudgmental*
5. *Service to Others*
6. *Are Humble*
7. *Are Honest, because liars cannot lead*
8. *Acquire Knowledge*
9. *Have High Morals*
10. *Leaders, Don't Complain*
11. *Cultivate Growth in Others*
12. Good *Health*

"The exertion of energy in facing and overcoming difficulty strengthens character. Each time we face Difficulty and use our faith in our Lord to overcome it, there is a reward. This reward gives us the incentive to try and try again."

--Honorable Minister Louis Farrakhan

Becoming a Well Made Man

"Leadership is not for the arrogant."

—Honorable Minister Louis Farrakhan

All real and true knowledge comes from (Allah) God. He is the Author of all knowledge. In the *Bible*, Solomon devises a curriculum by which we can learn to become like he is, he does not tell us to go to school; not Solomon. He did not tell us what books to read or what definitions to look up. He said if you wanna be as wise as I am, he said "go to the ant thou sluggard." The *Bible* records that Solomon said go to a little thing called the ant and consider her ways and be wise; which having no guide, overseer or ruler, provideth her meat in the summer and gathers 'her food in the harvest. What this means is that the ant is self-motivated. The ant has its own qualities built up in self where it knows how to listen to its own consciousness. It doesn't have a need of somebody outside to constantly pushing at it or driving it to achieve.

By studying the ant, we as men can grow beyond need of someone lording over us, beyond the need of somebody calling us to be responsive and responsible. We don't need someone before us when you learn the ant's way. As men we don't like doing what nobody tells us to do which is a direct result of Post Traumatic Slave Syndrome (PTSS) anytime we hear something like *'order, fall in, what's your ETA?, We need everybody to give. We need everybody to do.'* As soon as we hear that even though it's coming from one that looks just like us, we as men immediately have the subconscious image of Willie Lynch, John Hawkins or some other slave-master. Soon as somebody says that we *must do* or *should do* or we *need to do*, our response is *'I ain't doing nothing.'* We are people that don't want a guide, don't want a seer, don't want a leader but are most in need of somebody to help us out. This is why the world is so afraid of the Honorable Minister Louis Farrakhan. *He's a different breed of leader*. Outside of the Nation, every other leader that has come before has been a thief and a robber. They used the cause and condition of a people as a wave. They used an organization or a religion as a surfboard. With their goal being to continue to ride the wave of our wretched condition for their personal benefits. No surfer is looking for a little wave to ride. They are always trying to find a bigger wave. Anytime someone stands before us as men and wants to convince us to follow them as a so-called leader, know that unlike the Honorable Minister Louis Farrakhan they are not looking at solving problems, they are identifying our problems, beating us down so that they can derive some personal gain from our problems.

These fake leaders ride in on the condition of our suffering people. The make enough noise about it to get a audience with "Massa." Get into a back room at the big house, then cut a deal. They leave with a donation to their organization or themselves as individuals. Then you don't hear any more about the problem. That's Hush Money. That's selling out! What makes the Honorable Minister Louis Farrakhan different is that he's not a Negro leader, he's a ***divine leader***. He's not just a guide, he's a ***divine guide***. He's not a minister, he is the ***Honorable Minister***. He is a man chosen by God for us. He's not trying to lead you into worship of him. In every interaction private or public you have with this beautiful man, he's lifting you up and showing you a version of yourself that is greater than you thought of self and motivating you to become it. He speaks power to the powerful and teaches in a way that gives power to the powerless. We leave a lecture by him knowing that we got a defender. We leave knowing that we got somebody that can plead our case to the power structures of this world and we also leave with the internal ingredients that we need to be able to fight and change our own condition.

The job of a leader, the teacher, is to marry the mind, muscle and the money of a community together that the community can collectively produce something bigger than they can do on their own. This is the test of us as men, are we able to produce, from our combined mind and might, our own schools, our own restaurants, our own daycares, our own grocery stores? Do we really want our own farmland where we grow pure food for our families? Our own system of commerce? We will make our own environment wherein which we can take what comes out of self, creating an sustained environment where our children, women and girls can be safe and free to express themselves in a righteous environment that we control.

We must marry our might with knowledge and wisdom. The more knowledge we put in our mind, the higher we can "fly." Notice that a open book looks like a bird with its wings open. Why? Because knowledge raises you. The higher you are, the more you can see. The more you can see, the better the strategy and plan can be. Have you noticed that in most cities, the mayor's office is on the highest floor in the city building? At an apartment building, the penthouse suite is on the top floor. The presidential suite at a hotel is never on the first floor next to the gift shop, it's always at the top. There is even a saying about having the "bird's eye view." One with a bird's eye view sees more, sees further, sees with a panoramic view forward, backwards, right and left. The Minister has caused us to see and understand, that for every physical law in the universe, there is it's spiritual counterpart. Seeing forward is seeing future. Seeing backwards is seeing the past. We should reflect on the past to avoid being a repeat offender of same mistake, but not dwell on the past. One of the biggest impediments to change and ultimately to success, being unwilling to forgive ourselves for our own past. Allah says in the *Holy Qur'an* that He takes souls by night. And whoever the decree of death has not been decided for, He returns their soul. This means that, if you woke up, God still believes in you. Well if God believes in you, who are you to disbelieve in yourself. You have the ability, time, in spite of your sins, shortcomings and defects to be what Allah (God) brought you here to be.

Listen to this wisdom from the Honorable Minister Louis Farrakhan; he said, "What living organism moving forward and looking backwards {at the same time} can make progress?" Try it and you will absolutely run into something. You will not only hurt yourself but you may even kill yourself. Instinctively, anytime you are moving forward but looking backward, you move slower than you need to move to get from where you are to where you need to be. It's only a matter of time before the discouragement of moving slow and injuring yourself alone the journey will cause you to quit all together. Remember, our offspring are also watching….. Keep your eyes on the prize not your past.

In physics, there is an axiom that says, The whole is greater than the sum of it's parts. Each part brings it's on energy, space or power, but when they come together, their energy becomes synergy. They don't just add strength. They multiply strength. Now there also is a negative opposite force that can come into play. It's called antagonism. This is when the parts come together and weaken the energy and power of the parts. This can happen without us if we live in the prison of our personal past or are infected by the damnable diseases of envy or jealousy. The Honorable Minister Louis Farrakhan shared this about envy, it's effect, and it's cure at a meeting in February 2013 in Rosemont IL. He says, "The light that you have is gradually diminished in the one who envies. There are two things you can do to get under envy:

1. You are not a Muslim or righteous person until you for your brother what you want for yourself.

2. Work hard to discover your gift and you will never envy or hate another human being who is manifesting theirs.

Solomon, who is considered the wisest man of the Old Testament, was being questioned by those that admired him, on how they could become wise like him. Interestingly, Solomon didn't point them to a book to read or a course to be a part of. He pointed them to the ant. The ant is something to be studied, what's so powerful about this thing called the ant? The ant, according to its nature, has no envy or jealousy. No ant is aware of the big picture nor the assignments of the other ants. So they are never looking around asking, "why aren't they doing..." or, "how much longer do we have to...". They aren't concerned with what other ants are not doing. They have 100% focus on their specific assignment. There is no rugged individualism among them. The ants live in colonies only. Ants can't live by themselves. Two ants can't survive. They have to have a community in order for them to remain in existence.

To become a god, walking among men, we must study the ant. Prophet Muhammad (PBUH) said there's three things that you need to remain a Muslim: Allah (God), His Messenger and a community. In order to be a well made man, we must be connected to Allah (God) and His Christ, as well as the brotherhood and the sisterhood. The ant needs a community in order for it to live and so do we.

The ants are without the knowledge of personal pain. *They only recognize what hurts the group*. No matter what you do to stop them, the ant can't feel it. They don't feel it when you step on them. They don't feel pain period. Why, because in the feeling of personal pain, this emotion could stop you from becoming as great as you could become, from becoming a leader, to becoming a god. The Honorable Minister Louis Farrakhan is our example. He is a Believer and a *Well Made Man*. No matter what type or intensity of opposition comes His way, He calls on Allah (God) and goes forward, not looking back, but in the moment, filled with the spirit of Allah. And this is how we have to be as men. A Well Made Man is a man filled with the Spirit of God.

"You know that we are savages. So we got to be patient with our people. But brothers, you got to study. And the more you study the words, the teachings, the very spiritual roots of his Word and the program of the Honorable Elijah Muhammad, you grow into the mind of a Saviour. And when people see you coming, they act as though a Saviour has come into their midst."

—Honorable Minister Louis Farrakhan

Neighbor + Hood

"We need 10,000 fearless men to go into the Black community, stand between the guns of the gangs and then settle this with conflict resolution!"

—Honorable Minister Louis Farrakhan

The phrase 'concrete jungle 'has become an unfortunate description of the Black community in every city in the United States of America. When people refer to the Black community, very rarely do they say 'community 'or even 'neighborhood. 'In fact, when we refer to the area in any city where Black people are the dominant population, we don't even call it neighborhood, we just call it 'the hood'. Why do we just call it the hood? Because the concept and function of 'neighbor 'is the missing in the environment that we live in.

According to the dictionary, a jungle is an environment where wildlife rules, so it has been in the Black community. We have become like wildlife. The good thing is, that there is a formula, which has been worked in wildlife environments, that if we employ that same formula in the concrete jungle, we can reverse the reality that we live in today. Master Fard Muhammad said, We have been made other than our own selves. We are not by nature savage. We are not by nature unrighteous. Nature regulates our affairs from the inside out, but when one is made other than their own selves, they operate outside of their nature. When nature is turned off, we lose the capacity to self regulate. It is then that we need laws, rules, regulations, a exterior system to regulate our affairs. *The Restrictive Laws of Islam and the Guiding Rules of Conduct*, which are 16 laws and a supporting list of good manners that support good morals serves as a basis of the necessary exterior system that will regulate our affairs, recalibrate the Black man's mind and get us back into our nature. If you do not have a copy of *The Restrictive Law of Islam is Our Success* by the Honorable Minister Louis Farrakhan, go to store.finalcall.com and order it.

It is a fact, that good manners promote good morals. The more our manners are up, the easier it is for us to keep and obey the Laws of God. We cannot just be obedient to the statues. A statue is a law. In fact, this is why a fixed object, made like a person or an animal, is called a statue. Which is how the Law of God is. This is why when someone commits an infraction or violates one of the rules or the commandments, statues or laws of God, it's inappropriate to say that brother or sister "broke the law." They did not actually *break* the law. If they had actually broken the law, then after they violated the law then the law would in fact be less in importance. But the law is a statute. Whenever someone violates the law, they didn't break the law, the law broke them! The violator of law becomes of less value and importance not the law itself. In the *Holy Qur'an* 17:32 it reads, *And go not nigh(near) to fornication:* This provides us with a 'Discipline

Hack' if you will. It's a secret formula to keep you in accord with the law. "Go not near" In other words don't even go in the environment where you will be tempted to violate divine law. This is the great value of the *Rules of Conduct.* They keep us from even being in the proximity of wrong behavior.

One of the titles of Messengers and Prophets is a Reminder. Therefore, the *Holy Qur'an* and the *Bible*, which record the words and ways of them are also reminders. Re-Mind, the prefix Re- means to do again or put something back. The *Bible* and *Holy Qur'an* are putting truth and our innate natural way that we have forgotten back on our mind. The *Holy Qur'an* and *Bible* are really our nature on paper! We need them remind us of and to re-activate our divine nature. Before there was Christ as a character, we had Christ Consciousness. Before there was Muhammad the Man, we had the Muhammad Mind. Before there was Allah in person, we possessed an Allah Awareness. It's only when we stopped listening to this inner voice, this self-accusing spirit, this messenger of God within that their became a need for messengers without. We use to be able to hear God within and study nature without to make wise, divine, and correct decisions. The Honorable Minister Louis Farrakhan teaches us that we live in the very mind of God and that the universe is God's University. This is why the *Holy Qur'an* reminds us many times, "*there is a message in creation for those who believe, there's a message in creation for those who reflect, theres a message in creation for those who keep their duty.*" Even Solomon, the wisest man of the Old Testament, when he was being asked how to become wise. He didn't point his students to books, he said "study the ant". He pointed them to nature. By studying nature, we can learn brotherhood and sisterhood, parenting, optimal eating habits, business management, agriculture etc. The only difference between man and animal is that man has a free will and the ability to write and speak; other than that, man and animal are identical to one another.

In the *Holy Qur'an*, it says that we created all of the animals and all of the insects; listen to this, *in communities* like yourselves. So technically, when man is manifesting the supreme expression of self, we don't have to study the animals to learn how to be what we're supposed to be; they're supposed to be studying us. The *Holy Qur'an* has 114 chapters. Allah (God) revealed all of the words in the *Holy Qur'an*.

The second chapter of the *Holy Qur'an* is called The Cow. In fact, it's 1/15th of the entire book; the longest of all the chapters is Al Baqarah, The Cow. Why is it called The Cow? Because just as a cow has seven digestive systems, which purify all of the food it eats, to make the best food on the planet, when taken straight from the udder of a cow, pure raw milk. It is a perfect food for man. Milk, the *Holy Qur'an* says is a pure drink, for the drinker, and just as the cow has seven digestive systems that can take food from a corrupt world and turn it into a perfect food, so it is for a true Believer. If we are in the world but not of the world, we can get the best that this world has to offer and purify it through our seven digestive systems and make milk for our people: a perfect food.

Surah 16 is entitled *The Bee.* The Bee teaches brotherhood. The Bee teaches a high level of proper organization. In the beehive, the other bees always look out for the leadership. When you have a beehive, you have satellite hives and then you have a headquarters hive. The satellite hives make honey for the headquarters hive; so it is with human organization. The bees are special. They land on different flowers in different environments of different hues and colors; but when they land on each flower no matter what environment that they land on it can be in the ghetto or it can be under a gazebo, it doesn't make a difference. The bee lands on all the flowers, extracting pollen. Pollen is the best of each of the flowers that it lands on and it adds this to the best that it has within itself and the next thing we know, there is an integration of the best of the bees interior with the best from all the flowers, brought back to the hive.

Through working together in this process, the bees produce honey. Honey gives the eater energy, medicine, B vitamins and healing. And if we work in brotherhood, in unity, these same benefits will come to us. We are each a species of flower born in different environments, planted in different soils. We might be a different species of flower but we all have pollen in us. What would happen if every time we met a brother we didn't care about the negative of the brother. No, we would be giving to each brother we meet our very best. Give me your best young brother. Give me your best and I'll put my best with your best and give it to the world as honey. That's brotherhood.

In the 29th surah of the *Holy Qur'an*, is a perfect description or analogy of the concrete jungle. It is entitled *The Spider* and it opens up asking,

'Do men think that they will be left alone on saying they believe and will not be tried, when surely we tried those before you, so that we might know the truthful ones from those who are the liars.'

Allah (God) already knows the real from the fake, the true from the false, the liar from the honest one, and the real brother from the one that is a hypocrite. Allah (God) does not test us to prove to Him, but there's a god in us that is unaware of what we are truly made of. So Allah (God) begins to organize people, situations and circumstances to test us so that we will know how much god we possess.

"Good men, and good women, start by recognizing how insufficient we are, and how Great God Is. In the Muslim Prayer Service, you see us raise our hands near our head as if we are in an act of surrendering to Allah (God), and we say, Allahu Akbar, which means "God is Great." Not "I," but God is Great. Then, as we continue the prayer, the Muslim goes into a bend, where he says, "God is Great. Blessed is the Name of God, and surely God answers him who praises Him." But then the Muslim says even bending is not enough, so he prostrates himself, returning to the fetal position (sajdah) to remember that he was once in the womb, made from worthless water, and God brought him forth. So who are we that we should get carried away with ourselves? Humility is how you start making a few—just a few—good men.

Now, when we say a few good men, the word "few" means "not many; a small number; a minority group"—a select group. The word "good," according to Webster, means "suitable to a purpose." A lot of people are suitable for some purpose, and they are effective. They may be efficient. They may produce favorable results, and the results may be beneficial. But they are not yet a few good men, because "good" is not what we define. "Good" is what God defines.

The scripture teaches that "God is Good." Well, if God is Good, then it is only He Who sets The Standard, or gives the yardstick by which we measure what is good! Unfortunately, we don't use that yardstick, and that is why there are only a few."

—Honorable Minister Louis Farrakhan

Theology of Adversity

You were made to conquer whatever life presents. You did it as sperm, why do you think you can't do it now.

—Honorable Minister Louis Farrakhan

"Do men think that they will be left alone on saying, We believe, and will not be tried? And indeed We tried those before them, so Allah will certainly know those who are true and He will know the liars." ~*Holy Qur'an* 29:3-4 Of course Allah doesn't need trials to know who is true and who are the liars. He can read hearts. The Honorable Minister Louis Farrakhan teaches us that it's the God within that needs confirmation on who we are. So trial become the blessed opportunities to prove to self, that we are who we say we are. The *Holy Qur'an* teaches that trials purify. Here's a conversation the Devil is having with Allah in the *Holy Qur'an* Chapter 15:39-40 - He(Satan) said: My Lord, as Thou hast judged me erring, I shall certainly make (evil) fair-seeming to them on earth, and I shall cause them all to deviate, Except Thy servants from among them, the purified ones. Except the purified ones. Well if trials purify and Satan will get all except the purified ones, then trials purify us in a way that gives us spiritual immunity from Satan himself. So our spirit when adversity shows up, shouldn't be, "Why me?" It should be, "Try me!" Try me, so I know that I am what I say I am. Try me, so I can know how strong I am. Try me, so I can gain spiritual immunity from the Devils!

When we study the *Holy Qur'an*, we will learn that trials come from four places. Number one, the minute we make our mind up that we are willing to be a follower of a messenger of God, the world will test you. Why, because the ultimate aim of this world is to kill the messenger of God and the more valuable we are to the message and that messenger, the more opposition we will have raised up against us. If we didn't want to have enemies and we didn't want to be tested, why did we decide to become men of Righteousness and Conviction? Being a Well Made Man ain't the role for you if you are weak and cowardly. But, if you want to be a god and do the work of God and help the Messenger of God, then Allah (God) will protect you.

Allah (God) says that He will try us with something of fear, hunger, loss of property, loss of life and loss of money; the diminution of fruits. These are called preordained struggles. Whether you are in, out, believe, or don't believe anymore, active or inactive, you will be tested. Wouldn't it be better to take a test and be able to move closer to Allah (God) and enrich the brotherhood by your testimony of how Allah (God) brought you through, than to sit on the sidelines and complain and Facebook criticize?

On the third level, not only will we be tested by the preordained struggles, but Allah (God) says through Prophet Muhammad (PBUH) that when Allah (God) has predetermined a rank for His servant that that believer has not attained by the working of their own hands, uh oh, that's another way of saying there is no mystery god. Allah (God) says that He changes not the condition of a people until they change first change themselves. The Nooruddin translation says, in essence not only their condition must change but their "thoughts" and their "ways" must also change. The methodology, by which one changes their own condition, is that we as men must change what we do and what we think. And when we change what we do and what we think on a daily basis, then change will be caused in us and those around us. Allah (God) says if the Believer does not achieve the rank that was preordained for him, then He begins to afflict that Believer; through their children, their health or their wealth and He remains patient over that process until that servant becomes (submits) to what Allah (God) preordained for them to become.

Anytime that something is not going right, there is nobody to blame but self. 'Man I'm broke.' Why? 'I ain't working hard enough but I am working hard, but maybe I ain't working smart then.' No excuses. Something going wrong with self, ain't nobody responsible for it but me. I need to make some adjustments, modify time distribution, change my attitude, and the greatest fix I have ever discovered is asking myself this one question and answering with actions, "What has Allah asked me to do that I'm not doing?" Once I make my mind up to start making those prayers, etc. I change and things change. Part of being a weak man is blaming and complaining. Part of being a Well Made Man is taking full responsibility for self. Allah (God) says in Chapter 42:30 in the *Holy Qur'an*, "And whatever misfortune befalls you, it is on account of what your own hands have wrought.." Whatever means all, not some, but all of the misfortunes that befall man are on account of what man's own hands have wrought. In some way, our mixture of thoughts, words, and deeds birthed the circumstances of life. Sometimes we pray for things and forget that blessings have burden and rewards have responsibility. So Allah, ofttimes has to allow circumstances to present themselves to ensure that we are constitutionally fit to handle what we ask Him for.

Allah (God) tells us in Chapter 25:20 of the *Holy Qur'an*: "*And we make some of you a trial for others. Will you bear patiently?*" So the fourth category, by which trial comes, is by means of other people. There's some people no matter what you say they still will be in opposition. Sometimes those "who rub us the wrong way," can turn into rubbed the right way, if we handle the circumstances by bearing patiently and rise above emotions into the thinking of God, we come out of the encounter stronger, better, and wiser. Another way we are tried by means of others is looking to curry favor with others vs. pleasing Allah. Allah (God) wants to know 'do you want to please men or do you want to please Me?' 'Do you seek refuge in them or do you seek refuge in Me? 'The minute that we compromise our principles for the pleasing of a person, is the minute that we have officially lost our moral and masculine integrity. When you are loyal to principle and seek refuge in Allah (God), the person can test you all they want and it will have no effect. In fact Paul warns in scripture that a man should, 'Beware when all men speak well of you.' Something is very wrong with you if everybody likes you. Now, don't get me wrong, most people should like you. If you don't get along with nobody then that's not the other person, that's you. A brother told me once, "Brother look, I was at this one restaurant, man the waiter, man I had cuss the dude out." The next time I saw the same brother he said, "Yeah, I was at the shoe store getting these shoes, man they was sitting there talking crazy, man I cussed that dude out." I said brother, man "Every time you talk to me whether it's the gym, or the shoe store, or the restaurant, it's always about how you cussed somebody out." I said "let me ask you a question, do you know what's the common denominator in all these scenarios?" He said, "Cussing 'em all out." I said no, "YOU! Could it be that you might be the problem because? I went to the same restaurant and I go to the same gym and I ain't never cussed nobody out. Everything's good when I'm there, I don't understand what's happening with you."

We have to understand that we are our own worst enemy. In fact, if you were to sound out the word 'en e my 'it tells us where the real one is; en-e-my, inner-me. So, the spider is another lesson that has to be studied. While the bee teaches the building of brotherhood, and the proper structure of organization, the spider teaches us how an organization is broken up; how brotherhood is destroyed. In nature, you will find that there are 35,000 different species of spiders. They spin their webs in different kinds of locations. The universal rule is they love dark and dirty and cluttered spaces. They love the dark. So, the key to keeping a spider away is you gotta be clean. You gotta be organized and you gotta keep it bright with the lights on. The spirit is what makes the atmosphere light up in the mosque, not the recessed lights, not the track lights. When you contribute to the collective consciousness of the people's spirit, then love is in the atmosphere, joy is in the atmosphere — the lights are on.

Some spiders like being under the bridge. Some put a web right between two bushes, in the walkways every day. Just like there are spiders that like spinning webs in different kinds of environments, the fact that the surah called the spider opens up about the believer being tested tells us there are even spiders that like spinning webs in the church and mosque. Did you know that everybody that says "As-Salaam Alaikum ain't no Muslim and everybody that says "Praise the Lord" ain't actually with The Lord?" Did you know that there are agents that the government sends into the houses of God? Did you know that there's such a thing in the community called a hypocrite? A hypocrite is a voluntary agent doing the work and will of the enemy and not getting paid nothing; working for free. Hypocrite, hypo means secret. 'Crite 'means to criticize. So hypocrites are those that criticize others in secret. The minute that you are around people that always have something to say about this one or that one or elusively about leadership then you are looking at a hypocrite; someone criticizing in secret. A hypocrite is the devil's devil.

A hypocrite is Satan's spiritual counterpart. The enemy knows that they can't come in here so they have to find a Black body to put their mind into. It's a circle of brotherhood. And while the open enemies of the rise of our people are working on causing us to implode, the most damaging to the destruction of our circle is by explosion or matter and energy flying outward from within. In one of our lessons the question is asked, "Why did we run Yacub and his made devil from the Root of Civilization in the Holy City of Mecca, over the hot desert" on a westerly course making him "walk" "2,200 miles"? Why did we do that? Because they "started making trouble among the Righteous." What did they do? Told lies. What did they do, they "Accused the Righteous" causing them to "Fight." So, the goal of the hypocrite is to turn believers against believers, brothers against brothers. Why, because our unity is more powerful than a nuclear bomb. It's the job, of the bee hive. It's the job of the community to look out for the good of the whole.

Now those of us that are Muslims in the Nation of Islam, we are instructed to make all men and boys join the F.O.I., which means that we accept all individuals. They can come as they are but they can't stay as they are. If you had a legacy of being a gossiper, but joined the ranks, understand that we know that loose lips sink ships. This means that as men we can't let a disruptive force like that stay among us in the ranks unchecked. We cannot allow them to stay in the ranks of the righteous and keep gossiping. If you had a bad habit of always tearing other people down, trained into the crabs in the barrel mentality, you can't keep that. No, the *Holy Qur'an* says of the backbiter, the slanderer and the gossiper, it accuses them of being cannibals. Muhammad asked, 'Would you eat the flesh of your dead brother…? ' Those who are cannibals…The first thing that happens according to science is that the one who eats the flesh of one like them is that they go insane. At the end of the day, you might be criticizing, complaining, talking bad about, slandering and gossiping somebody else, but your own sanity is at stake. At a certain point, you will go crazy.

We must be aware of and beware of the spiders. The White man is a spider. They have caught us in a web. And we've been in here struggling inside the web trying to survive as a people in the web of America. They look at us and they see us selling dope to each other, getting tired; killing each other, getting tired; struggling to survive, getting tired. They wait til 'we're all worn out and then the spider comes out of the corner and walks up to us, when we are at our weakest stage, sticking a needle into the head of the insect (us). The spider then sends inside of the body of that insect a poisonous enzyme. This enzyme works to break down the interior, leaving the exterior intact. Then the spider sucks all the insides out of the insect, feeding off it, while killing the insect. Understand, the insect, the body (outer appearance) of the insect is present and looks as though life is present in the insect. But what we are really seeing is a shell that has an outside with no inside. They have us in this condition so that we will be attractive to other flies coming around and they will think that it's safe to land never knowing that it is a trap.

We have 46 million Black people caught up in the political, economic, educational, and religious web of the White man. Dead on the inside but we look good on the outside. We fresh to def. Can't nobody do hair like Black people do hair. Can't nobody dress like

Black people dress. Can't nobody fix up a car like Black people fix up a car. We know how to make the exterior look like we are good, but on the inside there's no knowledge in our head. There's no wisdom. There's no understanding. There's no science of life. There's no culture. There's no refinement. There's no diet where we know How to Eat to Live. We become exterior objects that are hollow on the inside. The White man has been like a spider to us.

The Honorable Minister Louis Farrakhan has given to us a mandate, as men to "Make our communities a safe and decent place to live." What this means is that the new code for us is not, once you 'get a lil money get out da hood. 'The new code must be, 'when you get some money fix the hood up. '

Do you know what you do to a Black child riding their bike down the street, in the ghetto and they ride pass a long row of houses and all they see is crabgrass, dandelions and trash. But when you have your family in the hood and you have taken the mandate of the Honorable Minister Louis Farrakhan as your personal responsibility, striving to take care of what Allah (God) has blessed you with, that same child rides past your home. That child looks inside of your yard and sees, healthy grass that almost looks like carpet. They see roses, birds of paradise, and sunflowers. They see a greenhouse and a hoop house in your backyard. Do you know what it does to the Black child riding their bike down the street? They stop and want to speak to you, 'Excuse me. Excuse me sir. What do you do for a living?' Do you know why they are really asking? What they are really saying to you is that, "what are we doing where we live? With old crabgrass and old dandelions, trash and chipped paint, it don't look like yours and I don't want to grow up and be like them, I want to grow up and be like you! What did you do? 'And when you begin to tell them that "I'm a Muslim, in the Nation of Islam, under the leadership of the Honorable Minister Louis Farrakhan" or "I'm a faith filled member of [whatever your house of worship is]", striving to live a righteous life. I'm actively engaged in wholesaling and retailing products. I have on the side some real estate and I'm not a slum landlord. I treat people the way I want to be treated. I'm an architect." When you began to tell him these things, next thing you know you see the little Black boy's eyes come open and they start riding they bike faster. Next thing you know that same child and his friends are at the library. What is he doing? He's at the library because he wants to be *A Well Made Man*!

"Black people are not balanced; nor is humanity in general. Allah (God) created us with a natural inclination towards Him. That inclination causes us to move in His direction from the very beginning of life to the end. But the journey to Allah (God) has been aborted because of Falsehood and the acceptance of Falsehood.

Our brains were created to <u>think right</u>. Falsehood, which is untruth or deception, produces a spiritual and chemical imbalance in the brain. And since the nine (9) systems of the human body all rely upon the brain, its imbalance results in a malfunctioning of the entire health system. Even though there may still be a regular heartbeat, normal blood pressure, etc. there is a very real dysfunction that ultimately shortens life—because Allah (God) intended for us not to be nearly balanced, but we are made to achieve exquisite balance."

—Honorable Minister Louis Farrakhan

Lessons from 'The Elephant'

On June 14, 2014 the news show *60 Minutes* ran a story detailing a study on what they classified as 'Rogue Elephants.' The 105th Surah of the *Holy Qur'an* is called The Elephant. Now when Allah (God) revealed the *Holy Qur'an* to Muhammad, He also revealed the names of the chapters. So there is revelation in the nature and function of the creatures Allah named the chapters after just like there is revelation in the verses of the chapters. The Elephant then, is a worthy study. *The Rogue Elephant Series* was filmed in South Africa. The elephants they spotlighted lived in Kruger Park and over time, Kruger Park began to overpopulate with elephants. In the warped mind of the White man, murder is always the solution for everything. In Kruger Park when the elephants began to overpopulate, they came up with a policy, '*kill the adults and spare the young.*' From helicopters, they started shooting all of the elder elephants, sparing the young ones. Then they used the helicopter to tranquilize the young and pick them up and carry them from Kruger Park all the way to a different park called Pilanesberg Park. They dropped the young off without a mother or father. After they dropped them off, in Pilanesberg Park they would observe them. What they noticed is that the dominant figure of the environment was the white rhino but as they came back to check on the baby elephants, they started seeing white rhinos dead everywhere.

Their original thought was that, 'Well, poachers must be killing the white rhino.' Poachers are those that kill for sport, taking the horns from the rhino for trophies or to sell them on the so-called "black-market." However, all the horns were still intact on the dead rhino's they found. Meaning, that it wasn't poachers doing the killings. The mystery was so great that scientists started secretly setting up cameras in the woods hoping to figure out what was really happing. What the scientists found was that these young elephants, taken originally Kruger Park, after their elders where killed and they were relocated to Pilanesberg Park, were in fact killing all the white rhinos. These same scientists classified the elephants that were killing the white rhinos, as a group of juvenile "*delinquents*" that had formed themselves into gangs. As they observed these young elephants over time, they realized that they were in fact getting more and more violent, more and more destructive. What they learned was that separating the young from their fathers and their mothers; there was no one there to teach the elephants proper elephant behavior. They did not learn their natural temperament. So because they did not have their natural guide, their natural mentor, their natural teacher, their mother and their father there to coach them along, then they began to pick up on the dominant figure of the environment that they lived in which was the white rhino.

These young elephants began to live other than their own selves. They started eating like the white rhino. They started becoming aggressive like the white rhino. They began fighting each other and even killing each other. Why? Because they were taken from their mother and their father to a strange land, dropped off in a strange land without no one to teach them their own way. They became a duplicate of the dominant figure in the society called the white rhino. Tell me that ain't happening in the concrete jungle with Black people!

We were taken from the Motherland, separated from our fathers, dropped off in a strange land and now because we had no one to teach us our natural temperament and behavior, we began to adopt the dominant personality of the main figure in the environment, not the white rhino but the White man. Today, we eat what White folks eat. We have sex like White folks have sex. We are low down like they are low down. We lie like they lie. We gamble like they gamble. We kill like they kill. We are other than our own selves.

These elephants, as it continued to go on, they began to look and found that because they were without the guidance and training of their mother and their father, they started having sex at an early age; but not sex for the purpose of producing new elephants, sex for recreation without responsibility. The natural pattern of an elephant is that they don't engage in a lot of recreational sex, they engage in what is called meaningful mating. But because they were not around the teachers, at a very young age they began to have a whole lot of sex. Guess what happened? As the same elephants began to produce children, the men or the males didn't know how to be a fathers because the only way that you can learn to be a father is if you can hear it spoken, or see it practiced. But, there were no adults there even to show the mother or female how to be a mother or the male how to be a father. Because the females did not know what it meant to be a mother, they hardly got up and moved from their home territory. In other words, they sat around a lot and the females, began to have obesity problems, bad health and were doing nothing to rear their children. The fathers or the males, because they didn't know what it meant to be a father, they were always out doing other things, never at home. When they were out, they were not hunting to find food; they were playing and being destructive. Sound a little bit like the concrete jungle don't it?

By being taught to be other than themselves, engaging in illicit sex at an early age, without any guidance on how to regulate their behavior or show them proper temperament and patience; they began to notice the prevalence of hasty and impatient decisions being made. The normally highly organized elephant society became very disorganized and destructive. These elephants began to attack and fight each other *all the time*. Ultimately, the scientists began to tranquilize them so that they could perform medical experiments on them. The results of these young juvenile elephant's experiments determined that they had more testosterone than any other elephant they had ever tested. Meaning that they would be more aggressive, more violent.

The scientists determined that they needed a solution to the problem. The solution was to come with a killer mindset, *'hunt em down, smoke em out'* and do what, *'kill em.'* At one point in the documentary Brothers, they showed how they found what they called the leader of the gang and they shot him with a tranquilizer. The first shot was to take him down so that they could give the death shot later; as soon as they shot him with the tranquilizer all the other elephants made a circle around him to protect him, putting their life on the line. You know what came next? You ain't killing mine. They were committed to their plan so they had one White boy, come out with a rifle and a stick *'haaaaa'*, yelling at the elephants. The elephant backed up, looked at the White boy with a stick and he took his trunk and went up into the tree and pulled down half the tree *'rooomp'*. White boy hurried up and got in the Winnebago but they wouldn't leave so they brought the helicopters in.

Helicopters were brought in because the elephants had learned over time to associate them with being where the snipers were, the elephants normally hear the helicopter and they run because they think they are about to be killed. When the helicopter came in all of the elephants scattered but there was one that refused to leave she was the blood sister of the leader who had been tranquilized. She stayed there on post, waiting until they brought the helicopter all the way down. This is how the Black woman has been for us. She's been there as our protector at all cost! Eventually, she left and they killed him. But understand that this is how the White man is working with us — daily. The White man is performing a magic trick on us. Magic is all about the sleight of hand. It's about having you focus consciously on one thing while they're doing something different that you can't even pick up with your conscious mind. What the White man has us doing allows him to be free to perform what they call *justifiable homicide*; he has us looking at the effect as the cause.

Black people are not the cause of the problems in our community; we are the effect of it. Victor Hugo said 140 years ago, that "If the soul is left in the darkness, sins will be committed but the guilty one is not the one that commits the sin; the real guilty one is the one that created the darkness.[1]"

Our enemy killed off the mothers and fathers of these young elephants dropped the children off in a strange land. Now these young ones are engaging in inappropriate behavior that makes them a threat to the environment and now the solution after they do that is they want to kill them off. It's a wicked death plan! The exact same plan that our open enemy has used on us. After they kidnapped us, killed our parents, dropped us off in America and now they come with a wicked death plan and policy called justifiable homicide! We are the effect but they are the real cause! These elephants, they were no real problem as long as all they were killing were white rhinos and each other; but when they started messing with the tourist revenue; by attacking whole buses filled with tourists. White folk's tourism revenue started dropping and that's when things changed. Their god is money. No, money is their God. When you look on your dollar and it says 'In God we trust, 'they not talking about the God we believe in. G-O-D is an acronym, it stands for Gold, Oil and Drugs; that's God to them. That's what they worship.

[1] Monseigneur Bienvenu in Les Miserables

This was such an issue, the lack of tourism revenue due to these "rouge elephants" that the scientists came up with a new plan. They decided to go back into Kruger Park and capture some of the adult elephants that were in Kruger Park where they first had killed most of them and carry them over in the helicopter and drop them off in Pilanesberg Park. This time they only took adult males that were biological brothers. They took the male elephants from Kruger, brought them to Pilanesberg and even though these same juveniles had been killing and maiming each other and the white rhinos, they dropped off a few adult males and within a 30 day cycle there were no more deaths. The women that were there, the female elephants, they began to get up and move around now. The female elephants began to care for the young and to teach them how to use their trunk to gather the water, how to hunt, how to feed. These same elephants stopped destroying the environment they lived in.

When the *real men* came back, when they had someone there that could be a standard-bearer. They then turned on the White folks and they started looking out for the babies. Turned on White folks but they looking out for their women now. Turned on White folks but they are raising their young males to become fathers and men. Turned on White folks but they are organized. Turned and made their neighborhoods a decent place to live! That's what they did. I'm saying to us, brothers: We have to return back to our homes and we have to operate in a way that we have so much wisdom, knowledge and understanding that it no longer takes a whole lot of talking; it just takes walking. The presence of a real man, that carries the proper atmosphere. We should be able to show up like the male elephant getting out of the helicopter and let everybody know *daddy's back*. Then we can make our neighborhood a clean, safe and decent place to live. The concrete jungle can become heaven right here on Earth.

"The Honorable Elijah Muhammad said put on a white shirt, and put on a tie, I don't care if you only have one suit, beloved. Let it be clean! Even if it is a mismatch; let it be clean! Go clean among your people. Because clean is the opposite of dirty. Dressed-up is the opposite of undressed. You are going to a savage people who are undressed and dirty and if you go clean and dressed up you are opposite them and it sets up an immediate attraction; for opposite attracts. All praise is due to Allah.

If you go out among them looking as wild and ugly and crazy-acting as they look, you repel because you look like they look. But if you come with a peaceful expression, if you come with a heart filled with love for your people, who have never been loved by anybody except God and His Apostle, then you come in the Spirit of a Saviour. You come in the spirit of a Redeemer. A Redeemer is one who is willing to pay a price to redeem someone or something that he loves. If we love our people, then we have come forward to pay whatever price is absolutely necessary to redeem all of our people from the grip of Satan.

We are Saviours. We are Redeemers. So we say in our prayer, "My prayer, my sacrifice, my life and my death is all for Allah." It is all for Allah. Well what do you mean it is all for Allah? It is all for His Will. What is His Will? His Will is that the dead must be raised to life. But how will the dead be raised? The Truth must be gotten to them. And how will the Truth be gotten to them? The Truth must be put in vessels that will carry it to the lost and found. Knock on their door with a friendly face: a face of a Saviour - alive and alert-knowing that his brother is a savage and is crazy-acting; and the Saviour knew that but He walked among us for three and one-half years: among a savage people. We weren't too filthy for Him to come among us, to knock on our door, to walk in and sell us silks and different things so He could get a chance to teach us of this amazing word that He Himself had brought to save us and redeem us from the clutches of a brutal beast.

You are a Saviour, Blackman. You are not a destroyer, you are a healer. You're not a killer, you're a Saviour. "Wait a minute now I'm getting in shape." Stay in shape, but hide your power. Stay in shape but don't parade power. Parade the fact that you are a Saviour of your people. Don't make your people afraid of you, make them come toward you. Be warm and friendly. You know. Be courteous to your people. Be loving and kind to them. Yes. That is what wins them because for four hundred years they have known nothing but people talking to them hard, talking to them mean.

You know that we are savages. So we got to be patient with our people. But brothers, you got to study. And the more you study the words, the teachings, the very spiritual roots of his Word and the program of the Honorable Elijah Muhammad, you grow into the mind of a Saviour. And when people see you coming, they act as though a Saviour has come into their midst."

--Honorable Minister Louis Farrakhan

'The Man'

"Allah always delivers His servants."

—Honorable Minister Louis Farrakhan

In the *Holy Qur'an*, the 76th Surah is entitled, *'The Man,'* not *'a man,'* but *'The Man.'* 'The 'is a definite article. 'The 'is the supreme example. '*The Man'*, 76th Surah, 76 trillion years, *'The Man'* is the Perfect Man, Master Fard Muhammad. Master Fard Muhammad came and He brought to birth a spiritual process called, the Nation of Islam in the West, which is a high-speed duplication process. Designed to do what it took Master Fard Muhammad 40 years to accomplish. It was designed to put Him on the screen as the Master Document, put Him as the Master Disc in the duplicator, so that the Honorable Elijah Muhammad, a specially prepared man, could type in, not just 5 or 10, but 40 million and hit 'enter.' And 40 million blank minded Black people could come through the process and come out a master and a God, like Master Fard Muhammad! So Surah(Chapter) 76 is entitled, *'The Man'*, but the last Surah(Chapter) of the *Holy Qur'an* is titled the *'The Men'* which means that this one perfect man has now duplicated Himself and made a whole nation of gods.

When Allah (God) has decreed a certain rank, how do you know, how do we discern, that we are members of that elite group that Allah (God) has decreed a certain rank for? We discern it by knowing that Allah (God) could have picked anybody, any group geographically located on the planet, but He picked us, He specifically chose us.

When Master Fard Muhammad picked us, according to the Most Honorable Elijah Muhammad, *He handpicked each one of us.* This means He knew what some of us had smoked. He knew who we had lied to. He knew where we had been and what we had done and with whom we did it with. Yet, regardless to the mistakes and the errors, regardless to the lack of money that we thought we did not have or the perfect upbringing that we wish we would have had, He chose us. He chose us above the other 7 billion people on the Planet; not because we had more money than the next man did or because we looked better than the next man did. Not because we had a better upbringing than the next man did, but we had the quality of the heart, that Master Fard Muhammad was looking for to complete the process of making gods. Making gods out of men in the short period of time in which He had to work. We are the ones that had a 'rank 'decreed upon us before we even came into existence.

When the Son of Man was speaking to the bones and God told him, 'stop speaking to the bones, 'since they would not stand up and unite, God instructed the Son of Man to start speaking to the winds. To whip the winds up so that the winds would in fact whip them into shape. The goal of the Son of Man was not for those men to become an exceedingly great choir or an exceedingly great committee or an exceedingly great club. His goal was that they stand up, unite, and become an exceedingly great *Army. The goal of God for the Blackman is that we become the Army of Allah (God).* In the *Holy Qur'an*, Allah (God) uses terms: military terms or language in some areas. For example, the 33rd Surah of the *Holy Qur'an* is entitled "*The Allies*," military language. The 37th Surah is entitled "*Those Ranging in Ranks*," military language. The 39th Surah is entitled "*The Companies*," military language. The Most Honorable Elijah Muhammad, commanded those of us who are Registered Members of the Nation of Islam, to go among the men and boys in the neighborhoods and out in the highways and byways with the expressed goal to "Make all men and boys join the F.O.I." Not join, in order to be a part of a ministry, become a professional seat occupier, or become another stat on the books so it looks as though we are just fattening up our ranks. The Honorable Elijah Muhammad said after you make all men and boys join the F.O.I. he then said to, "Train them fast."

The reality is that when we are in the process of receiving; per the Honorable Elijah Muhammad's instructions, 'fast training 'some of us will get, not kinda or partly, but *absolutely* offended every now and then. Somebody may cuss at us every now and then. Somebody might rub us the wrong way every now and then, because we are trying to get something done fast. You don't always have a lot of time to sit around pontificating, negotiating, formally having this soft conversation over a cup of coffee with three cubes of sugar and a lemon bar. When you are training somebody fast, every now and then it's gotta be a *snap*, a *pop*, that *hear*, that *obey* because this fast process is designed to make them and make us into an exceedingly great Army of Allah (God). Understand that we are being trained to become brave fighters and we are not looking for everything to be 'honkey dory'. We are not looking for everybody to be nice. Hell, if you want that, get married. But brotherly love is not 'otherly 'love and 'otherly 'love is not among the *Well Made Man* description. The True and Living God don't raise no punks, no sissies, no faggots and no chumps. He makes MEN. Men love their brothers as their brothers and men love women as their mates.

The expressed goal of God in the *Bible* is for us to become an exceedingly great army, if the Most Honorable Elijah Muhammad says that His goal us as men. is that we become brave fighters, if you don't like fighting you are in the wrong mission. Maybe somebody didn't tell it. But I'm telling you now, that if you don't want to get shot at one day, you in the wrong mission. If you don't want to put your life on the line for the Messenger of God and the Message of God, you in the wrong mission. The Honorable Elijah Muhammad teaches us, that when the time to establish justice comes, there are three responses: The best response is that we raise our hands? Now we kill no one whom Allah has not ordered to be killed and even though we want to raise our hand, Allah (God) tells us in the *Holy Qur'an* that, "Fighting is enjoined on you though it is disliked by you." Allah (God) says, "And it may be that you dislike a thing while it is good for you. And it may be that you love a thing while it is yet evil for you."

The *Holy Qur'an*, then gives guidance on fighting, it says in Surah 2:178 that retaliation is prescribed. There are only three things in the

Holy Qur'an that are prescribed. What is a prescription? A prescription is a certain dosage of medicine designed to heal a condition. Prayer is prescribed. Fasting is prescribed. Along with prayer and fasting, is retaliation, which is also prescribed. In the same way that we can receive a spiritual healing from prayer, spiritual and physical detoxification from fasting, we can also get our mind and our heart and our being rejuvenated, revitalized when we make up in our mind to retaliate against our enemy when Allah (God) gives us the command.

Allah (God) also teaches us in the next verse (179) that, "Surely there is life in retaliation." So if there is life in retaliation and for every action there is an equal and opposite reaction, for those that don't want to be soldiers, for those that don't like military training, for those that don't want to become united and stand up, becoming *A Well Made Man* is in your destiny. It is not just good enough to come together. Brothers we got to stand up. In order to become a rank we have to live according to the Law of God. We can't come together in brotherhood if we are going to steal from a brother when the brother isn't looking. We can't come together in a bond of brotherhood if we're going to try to molest our brother's daughter. No man in his right mind would join on if someone is going to be looking at his wife whenever he's not around. A man in the brotherhood wants to know, that the brotherhood that he joined on with, that should he die on the battlefield, that my brother in the ranks, that loved me as their brother, will cover down on my family. That they will pool their resources and will provide for my family and that the brotherhood will want for my son and my daughter that which they want for their own sons and daughters. Without a united brotherhood, we are not a true Army of Allah, we cannot call ourselves *A Well Made Man* until and unless we want for our brother, what we want for ourselves.

"Everything in Creation is a manifestation of the Will of God. All of Creation expresses the Attributes or Characteristics of this Mighty Being, The Originator of the Heavens and the Earth. But the Will of God is the Power behind the throne. The Will of God is the Power behind the Universe; its creation, its maintenance and its sustenance.

—Honorable Minister Louis Farrakhan

Divine Unity

"Once you see what your unity can produce, then that victory will cause you to want to stay in unity for the next level of this struggle."

—Honorable Minister Louis Farrakhan

One area, which has been gravely misunderstood by us as men, is that the *Holy Qur'an* is a book that makes clear distinctions. One of those critical distinctions is in the types of unity that Allah (God) desires. The *Holy Qur'an* does not speak of regular unity or the type of unity that some of us found in this worlds military; it speaks about what it calls *Divine Unity*. The unity found in this world's military is a unity of action — there is the enemy, get the enemy. The Divine Unity of Brotherhood, extends beyond the battlefield. I see you as my brother, not born of my mother but born from the mind of Allah (God). We share the vision of the mission to redeem and restore our people and we are willing to sacrifice all that we have to bring that vision of a world built on the principles of freedom, justice and equality into fruition. We unite in Divine Unity when we hear and obey the General before us as he leads us through the valley of the shadow of death, successfully.

We learn from the Law of Cause and Effect that for every action, there is an equal and an opposite reaction. We get life from retaliation, and we get death when we punk out. The less we are willing to put our hands out there to build something that will stand against what we believe is wrong, the less that we are willing to speak out against the injustices being done to our people daily, the less we are willing to boycott in this world, the more we invite death into our own personal lives. Whenever we retaliate in accordance with boycotting, speaking against and raising our hands to build something for self, the more life comes into our life.

Why should we be afraid to fight? In the Nation of Islam we say that Allah (God) intervened in our affairs… When we say that Allah (God) came and intervened in our affairs. If Allah (God), Himself, has come to intervene in our affairs, this means He, Personally, has come to be with us in every challenge that we will face. Romans 8:31 says, If God be for you, who can be against you? The answer is, anybody, but they are wasting their time. You have the Supreme Being, the Creator, the All Knowing, Omnipotent, and All Powerful with you. They can't defeat you! This is the reason why, if we are mature, we will stop talking about what the hypocrite is doing, what the agent is doing, what the disbelievers are doing, what the weak ones are doing, what the laborers are not doing! Stop talking like that! To hell with Homeland Security, to hell with the FBI, the CIA and the ATF, to hell with the United States government, to hell with the Jews and the Zionists who have been working against us ever since our conception! We have a goal. A goal to build a Nation and when men come together to set a common goal, there's only four components present when a goal has been set; that is the person that set the goal, the goal, the forces working against them and the forces that are backing them up.

There are things working against us but all they are; are forces that are trying to keep us from achieving the goal. But my question is:

Brothers, who do we have backing us up? We've got GOD! In addition, with His Christ and Servant; who are all more powerful than all the forces of evil that are working against us, then they absolutely will neutralize and nullify all our enemies.

Brothers, there is nothing standing between us and the building of a successful business; nothing between us and opening up a grocery store. Nothing between us and buying an apartment building. Nothing between us and getting our farmland. Nothing between us and opening up a strip mall. Nothing between us and saving our people. Nothing between us and building our nation, but you and me and ourselves. Because the God and His Christ are handling everything that is working against our rise. All we have to worry about is what we are going to do. For we said, when we committed to become a member of the Army of Allah (God) — that we wanted to get up off our behind and go into the field and conquer the world like the Honorable Minister Louis Farrakhan. Nothing is stopping us but ourselves.

I recently read a book written by a man named Eliyahu Goldratt called *Goals*. In this book, Goldratt expounds on something called the 'Theory of Constraints. 'He considers the Theory of Constraints to be factors in between you and your goals that you determine to achieve. The factors that stop us from achieving the goal(s) as fast as we would like to are called constraints. Through Goldratt's research, he found that after interviewing people who expressed that they had a goal but didn't complete it, did complete it or completed it late. That 20% of the constraints, or the factors that stopped the individual or slowed them down from completing their goal, were from *other people or exterior circumstances*. The other 80% of all constraints that slowed the individuals down or stopped them from achieving their goal(s) came from within themselves as *artificial mental concepts, born out of fear and doubt in self.* What Goldratt expressed in a scientific way is what the Honorable Elijah Muhammad said, *"We got to get our own foot out of the way of our salvation."* Nothing is stopping us but ourselves because the God is possessor of power over all things, circumstances and events and absolutely has the Power to nullify everything that is in the way of us achieving our goals both personally and collectively.

This is the reason why being invited to become *A Well Made Man*, being invited to training, being in the classroom of God training to become a god and a brave fighter is so critical. It is something that we should be attracted to and energized by because Allah (God) promises us that He is going to help us. The 110th Surah of the *Holy Qur'an* is entitled "*The Help*" in this Surah, Allah (God) reveals that, "*When*," Let me take a moment to point out that it does not say 'if'. It says, "*When Allah's help*," so this means that He is coming, and *when* Allah's (God's) help comes! Allah's (God's) help is present among us. And what is the third part of Allah's help? '*Victory comes and thou seest men entering the religion of Allah in companies.*' This means whole sets of Crips, whole sets of Bloods, whole sets of Black Panthers, whole sets of Five Percenters (NGE's), whole sets of Moors, whole groups of Christians coming into the ranks of the Righteous, in companies, *"celebrating the praise of thy Lord and ask for His protection."*

What does Allah's help look like? In Surah 3:124 and 125, *"When thou didst say to the believers: Does it not suffice you that your Lord should help you with three thousand angels sent down?"* Now this does not mean that no angels with no wings will be sweeping down. This is not clear (see through) spirits coming to help us out. But an angel is a force of nature. An angel is an attribute of Allah (God). In the *Holy Qur'an* Surah 2:30, when Allah (God) said to the angels to bow down to Adam, and all of them did except for one, Iblis, these the Honorable Minister Louis Farrakhan teaches us were the attributes of Allah (God) that are being brought into submission to that 100th attribute which is Allah, Himself. So these attributes or these angels are forces within our own being. Allah (God) says if this does not suffice you that I'm helping, then I will send you three thousand angels, sent down. This does not mean that the ghosts are coming but what it means is that we would have the power in our individual constitution as if we've got three thousand angels working to full capacity in our being to achieve whatever we got in front of us. That's a pretty good verse. Allah (God) goes on to say despite that, this is just the reward for somebody that is just a Believer, because there are different categories of Muslims.

There are in fact three categories of Muslims. The basic category of a Muslim is a *Believer*. The *Holy Qur'an* speaks about another class, the *steadfast*. Then there is an elite class, the *foremost*. The only thing that separates these three classes is the degree of sacrifice of the individual for the good of the common whole or the common cause. The steadfast are those that do more and give more for the good of the whole and the foremost do more than the steadfast. The Believer, just on that level there expression and actions are that, *'I have the agreement and concept in my mind that Allah did appear in the Person of Master Fard Muhammad. The Honorable Elijah Muhammad is His Christ and the Honorable Minister Louis Farrakhan is their divine reminder.'* I believe. Just on that level of faith, there's three thousand angels sent down. For the next level, the steadfast soldiers. *"Yeah, if you are steadfast and keep your duty and they come upon you in a headlong manner, your Lord will assist you..."* This is what God's help looks like, Allah (God) will assist you "*with five thousand havoc making angels.*" Understand that these are not no regular angels. These are *havoc making angels*.

Brothers, do you remember that back in the day, we always had two classes of comrades or homies when we were in the streets? One class of people we had, if we needed them to come ride with us somewhere, we had to explain, "Look, so and so and them did such and such and so and so and I got the facts on such and such. I need you to go with me real fast." Ya'll remember they was the ones that want to ask questions and needed evidence. Then in the hood, there was always, in our circle, a havoc making Negro. This was the type of soldier we didn't have to do no explaining to. All we had to do was just say, "Look, bring that stuff. I'll be there in five minutes" And the response was always, "Sweet, meet me at such and such." He ain't asking no questions. He don't need no justification — havoc making Negro. This is the type that Allah (God) will send to our aide when the time comes — havoc making Negro Angels.

Brothers, bottom line is this: ***We've got too many citizens and not enough soldiers.*** Understand this ain't that kind of work. We don't have enough people yet to have people watching the news while we out on the battlefield! We don't have enough people yet to have you working the computer while we out on the battlefield. We are only a few good men right now and we need all hands on deck and everybody on the front line and not just a citizen of our Black Nation. We need soldiers in this Nation!

My brothers, let us remember that it is an honor, a privilege, that we should always thank Allah (God) for allowing us to be a student, a servant and a soldier in the Army of Allah.. Let us all pray to Allah (God) that we come together in a true bond of everlasting and real Brotherhood, for the time dictates the agenda.

Our mandate, from the Honorable Minister Louis Farrakhan is and will continue to be,

*"Make **our** communities safe and decent places to live."*

We are the men of God, we are *Well Made Men*! We Can! We Must! We Will!

How to Love a Black Woman

"Nature has placed in a woman a demand from the man and nature has placed in man a demand from the woman. Her demands has to be met before our demand can be met by her. You cannot expect a woman to give you what you demand, if you in the 1st place don't give her what her nature demands. Her nature demands a man to maintain, to uplift, to help to guide, to be a provider for and a protector of. And what you get in return for being a man is what God put in every woman, the consolation, the care, the love, that makes a man willing to go out and work the field or fight the Enemy to come back home."

—Honorable Minister Louis Farrakhan

"The process of marriage begins first with a natural attraction to some physical characteristics of the male and the female which please each other. This natural attraction then leads to a desire to be closer to that person whom we are attracted to, which leads to communication to get to know each other beyond the physical points of attraction."

—Honorable Minister Louis Farrakhan

The very best scholars and theologians have tried to define what love really is, and though they have made some admirable attempts, truthfully, they have all fallen short. Usually, they come to an agreement on a definition of the word love admitting that in truth they are still ignorant to the true substance of love. The Honorable Minister Louis Farrakhan teaches that music is the universal language of a people. When a person or scholar wants to learn what the dominate idea or philosophy of a particular group of people is, they study the lyrics of their songs. For example, if you want to know the dominate idea and philosophy of the Chinese people, listen to the music the Chinese people create. If you ever want to know what is the dominate idea and philosophy of the people of Saudi Arabia is, again, listen to the lyrics found in the music, in particular the most popular music.

When the world listens to the music of the Black man and woman of North America, what do our lyrics tell them about the dominate idea and philosophy of the so-called Negro mind? More importantly, what do our songs tell us about the way we think and operate? Inside of our music, when we are talking about the subject of love, it is clear that we have the definition of love all twisted up. We say love when we are actually talking about lust. We say love when we are actually talking about infatuation. We say love when we are actually talking about basic carnal (sexual) attraction. However, love is not some carnal attraction or some physical thing. Love is not lust. Love is not infatuation. You cannot fall into love. The *Bible* says, "God is Love." Well, if 'God is Love,' and 'God is the Most-High God,' how does one fall into it? We must come up into love, God is Love, and pure Love is God then, God is the Most-High expression of everything including love!

One of our great contemporary musical artists, Musiq Soul Child, had a very popular song several years ago. In the song he sang, "Love, so many people use your name in vain." Tina Turner, after enduring 16 years of abuse at the hands of her husband, Ike Turner, sang with great passion. 'What's Love got to do with It? What is love but a second hand emotion? Who needs a heart, when a heart can be broken?' In this modern time sisters, if a brother is asked does he love you? The brother will say if he is truthful, that he only loves you partly. He will tell you, as Drake said in his song, he "only loves his bed and his mama, I'm sorry." Then the day comes and you finally get a good look at how crazy his mama is and how broke down that little raggedy twin size bed he has been sleeping in is, you start saying, 'Wait, if you only love your momma and you only love your bed then what am I to you actually?'

If music is the universal language of a people that allows you to know the dominate philosophy and ideas ruling the peoples thinking and dictating their actions; then when we listen to the lyrics of our music as a people, it becomes very obvious, that Black men do not really know how to love a Black woman and somebody has to teach us! Who will teach us? One that has been raised by God to teach us the meaning of love, the proper application of love and how to love in accordance with God's way.

A quick Google search using the word relationships will return over 380,000 books on relationships usually with some real sophisticated or slick titles. What is most striking is that if you notice, out of 380,000 books on relationships, there were two books missing that should have been at the very top of the list. The *Bible* and the *Holy Qur'an*! All empirical data but no spiritual wisdom. Yet the first institution created by God, according to the scripture, was not the church, Mosque, or school, it was the institution of marriage. Genesis 2:18 (KJV) says, "*And the LORD God said, It is not good that the man should be alone; I will make him an help meet for him*." Help Meet, not Help "Meat". It is no question that men are more physical than women are. Men are more attracted to the female anatomy than women are attracted to the male anatomy. Allah in the *Holy Qur'an* calls the female's body parts "her adornments." Base word of adornments is adore. Adore means, to regard with the utmost esteem, love, and respect; honor; to like or admire very much. However, we must remember as men that marriage is called a sacred union, covenant connection, and holy matrimony. These are all spiritual terms, letting us know that the primary traits and characteristics we should be looking for in a woman to see if she is compatible are spiritual and mental above the physical. You can include the physical, but they should be at the bottom of your list. The Honorable Minister Louis Farrakhan asked this, "Have you noticed that rich white folks marry Rich white folks? We mate from the navel down. White people mate from the neck up."

Here are ten Spiritual traits in the *Holy Qur'an* we should be looking for to determine compatibility. *Holy Qur'an* 33:35 "Surely the men who submit and the women who submit, and the believing men and the believing women, and the obeying men and the obeying women, and the truthful men and the truthful women, and the patient men and the patient women, and the humble men and the humble women, and the charitable men and the charitable women, and the fasting men and the fasting women, and the men who guard their chastity and the women who guard, and the men who remember Allah much and women who remember — Allah has prepared for them forgiveness and a mighty reward."

Add your personality traits you like, then your physical traits. If the woman you are considering meets up to 70% of your ideal woman description, compatibility is present, so teaches the Honorable Minister Louis Farrakhan. If you marry a woman with less than 70% already present, you won't have a partner, you will have a project! You don't want a project. You want a partner, a helpmeet to help you with projects not be one herself. And the LORD God said, It is not good that the man should be alone; I will make him an help meet for him. Not good for man to be alone. Not good for man to be alone? Why?

Before we were kidnapped, Caucasianized and Westernized, the Black Family was our Power base! When Napoleon was hired in 1798 to destroy all images of black excellence in the temples, libraries and pyramids of Egypt. After Napoleon finished destroying the great image of the Black man's greatness, the Sphinx. A body of a lion, with the head of a Black man. Written at the base are the Arabic words, Abu El Howl, which means father of everything. He trained his cannons and blew off the nose and the lips because they verified that the head on this lions was a Black man. He and the white rulers who hired him did not want us get informed by way of image association, "if the lion is the king of the jungle and my ancestors put my head on the body of a lion, maybe they are trying to tell me that I'm the king of the planet and the father of everything! Can't make a slave out of a man with that thought process at the front of his mind. Then Napoleon went inside and noticed that every time he seen a image of the great gods and warriors of our people, thud always had their queens right by their side. Wherever you seen Osiris, Isis was right by his side. When you saw Osau, Ahset was right by his side.

When you saw Olefoon, Illedah was right by his side. This verifies and modifies the old saying, "behind every strong man there is a strong woman. No! Beside every strong man has always been a strong woman! There are a few observations we can extract from what our ancestors left on the walls of the pyramid Giza.

1. No men with men
2. They were married, no boyfriend and girl-friending.
3. All of the great Black men were with a great black woman.

The Most Honorable Elijah Muhammad said, "The only heaven for a Black man is found in a Black woman." When marriage is done right, your home becomes a spiritual recharge center where you can unplug from this wicked, no good, white supremacist world, and come home and plug up to a pure source of level that will give you peace and power! Your mate's spirit should uplift you. Her love should ease your mind. Their Intelligence should help you think deeper. Their Passion should inspire you. Your mate should help you evolve, and if they don't help you evolve, you should not be involved.

I hope these few paragraphs have provided why to be married and how to choose the one. Now we want to tackle the "How" to love a Black woman.

In the *Bible*, in the book of Ephesians, there are gender specific commands from the mind of God. Two different actions to that allow the man to get the best out of his woman and vice versa. It is written in Ephesians 5:33(NIV)

"…each one of you also must love his wife as he loves himself, and the wife must respect her husband." For her to get the best out of man she must use "respect" and honor but for the man to get the best out of his woman, he must "love" her. I know what you are saying, "but it was Aretha Franklin that sang the hit RESPECT.... This is true, but before it was released by Aretha Franklin in 1967. Ottis Redding wrote and released it on August 15, 1965. When questioned, Ottis Redding said the song was from him to his wife. If Aretha Franklin would have wrote the song from her nature, it would have LOVE.

In a 2012 Study on the Today Show. Women all over the world were interviewed and asked, "what are you looking for in a man?" After distilling the feedback, they came up with four universal desires women had for their ideal man.

LOYALTY- There is great infidelity insecurity in women. Most women are one-man women, but we have not been one-woman men. Allah (God) in the *Holy Qur'an* and *Bible* says, it is the nature and divine duty of a man to maintain, protect and provide for his family. All these acts produce security. Security is what nature demands in a woman from a man. Infidelity creates the greatest insecurity in a relationship. How can you be loyal? Follow the golden rule. Practice in all activity with the opposite sex, Do unto your wife what you want your wife to do unto you.

Security doesn't just come from paying the bills. Security comes when you love her out loud, come home every night, do not cheat, and spoil her just because.

To help add a level of security that curbs the enthusiasm of other women, where a wedding ring. A wedding ring is a sign, commercial, advertisement to others and a Reminder to self.

LABOR- Women are attracted to, turned on by and kept on by a hard working man! A man has to be a Hunter, Worker, Doer, Go Getter and a go Giver. When a man is in love with a woman, her needs become his goals. A real man gets more joy out of happiness of his wife and children receiving from him, than getting anything for himself.

LOVE- The 1st rule of Love is say it often to your wife. In fact, there are three sets of words that can instantly make a woman smile.

Try them with sincerity and at the right time. What are the three statements that touch a woman's heart?

I Love you.

I miss you.

You are beautiful.

Note: After saying I Love you, now we have to demonstrate it. Believe it or not, love isn't as expensive as we think. These are simple, cost less expressions of love that waters a woman's soil.

Holding her hand and holding her hand in the public. In the public, doesn't just say I love you, but also says "I like you" and I want everyone to know) -

Go on walks with her. Show affection without sex. Have date nights. Give spontaneous gifts (wants not needs) don't gift her windshield wipers are dishwashing liquid, get her something she likes and has expressed she wants. Do you want to be all the way up? The Honorable Minister Louis Farrakhan said, "Love anticipates need." Take care of some of her household responsibilities without her asking or knowing.

LAUGHTER - The women interviewed unanimously said that a sense of humor is paramount in a man. A Sense of humor is a sense of security. Sense of humor is a sense of strength. Sense of humor is a sense of faith. A woman wants to know, in the midst of turmoil and trial that everything is going to be all right. She wants to know that her man is a warrior, not a worrier and that you have everything locked down and secure. A soldier can smile and still be in a state of readiness for whatever!

LISTEN - Men *think* through their problems; however, women *talk* through their problems. A man has to be a good listener. To be a good listener, one has to give undivided attention to what is being said, put yourself in the other person's position, and be a positive soundboard for what is being said. Provide east ways to resolve whatever is being discussed and volunteer to be in unity with her in the subject of concern.

Loyalty, Love, Labor, Laughter, Listen and there is one more they missed…

The Honorable Minister Louis Farrakhan said, "*brothers, to be the head, you have to have a head.*"

"AN IGNORANT MAN CAN NEVER BE A GOOD HUSBAND. No man can be a supporter of a woman just with finance. It takes knowledge to support a woman. Finance can keep her up physically but knowledge can keep her up mentally and spiritually."

So we have to be

Loyal, a laborer, listen, love, laugh with AND *LEARNED*.

A WELL MADE MAN

INDEX

About The Author

Brother Nuri Muhammad, Student Minister of the Honorable Minister Louis Farrakhan, Author, Activist, Mentor, and Entrepreneur.

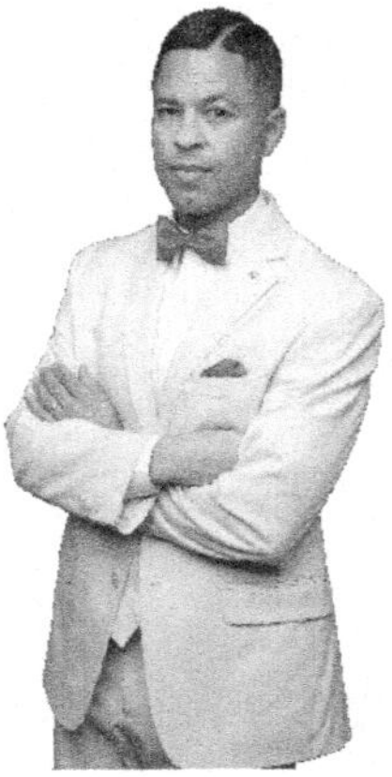

Brother Nuri is known for messages that have a bal mix of inspiration and information, which has mad one the most sought after speakers in the cour Whether it is a high school, church, college, prisc banquet or conference, his gift to collaborat scripture, science, and history in a user friendly way has him delivering 100s of messages a year in the United States and abroad. He is the author of six books, **Before You Say I Do, After You Say Do, Let this Mind Be In You, The 7 Jewels (God, The Black Woman: The 2nd Self of Go(and A Well Made Man**. Three of which are best sellers on Amazon Books. Excerpts of his speeches have been used in the songs of several major recording artists. Bro. Nuri also released his own album titled **The Black Excellence Manifesto Vol. 1**. A rhythm of truth project that mixes Bro. Nuri's lecture excerpts with Hip Hop and R&B artists laying tracks on 9 critical subjects of Black Excellence.

Nuri Muhammad has appeared on **The Breakfast Club** with Charlamagne the God, DJ. Envy, and Angela Yee, **The Daily Show with Trevor Noah, Revolt TV, Vlad TV** with DJ Vlad**, Ebro in the morning on Hot 97, and The Joe Budden Podcast.**

In addition to the National and International contributions he makes, Bro. Nuri takes great pride in being the Student Minister of Muhammad Mosque #74 in Indianapolis. This state of the art facility, which houses the Mosque, Classrooms, and two restaurants (Eat to Live Cafe and Always Bean). It is affectionately called "the miracle on 38th street" because it was purchased by young Black people, designed by Black architects, and renovated by all Black construction. The multimillion dollar complex is owned by the Mosque #74 community completely debt free.

NuriMuhammad.com

Made in the USA
Monee, IL
21 July 2024

62400918R10089